Paedophiles, Child Abuse and the Internet

A practical guide to identification, action and prevention

Adrian Powell
Child Protection, Paedophiliac Sex Offender Identification and Risk Management Professional

Radcliffe Publishing
Oxford • New York

Radcliffe Publishing Ltd
18 Marcham Road
Abingdon
Oxon OX14 1AA
United Kingdom

www.radcliffe-oxford.com
Electronic catalogue and worldwide online ordering facility.

British Library Cataloguing in Publication Data

A catalogue record for this book is available from the British Library.

ISBN: 978 1 85775 774 3

Typeset by Aarontype Ltd, Easton, Bristol
Printed and bound by TJI Digital, Padstow, Cornwall

This book is dedicated to Aimee and Thomas.

And to children who are suffering and have suffered child abuse
and those who still carry the scars.

Every one of them has been my inspiration.

Contents

Preface

Why this guide was written

After receiving a few snippets of information, making a few telephone calls and completing a little research, I identified a smartly dressed, well-mannered and nicely spoken, intelligent man who had obviously benefited from a sound education. He appeared as a respected pillar of our society. I shall refer to this man as Gerald.

I had, by that time, completed many years of work identifying, risk assessing and disrupting what the general public, the media and most professionals call 'paedophiles'. I had carried out this work alongside social workers, health professionals, police officers, probation officers, custom officers, doctors, mental health workers, psychologists, and professionals and volunteers within numerous child protection charity groups. Individuals like Gerald were familiar to me and establishing his activities was my primary role.

I discovered that for more than three years Gerald, a single and childless man in his fifties, had been attending his local swimming pool every week during the 'children and parent' sessions. Gerald would follow children around the pool, invite himself to play in their games and remain in the communal changing area for far longer than was ever necessary. He had aroused the suspicions of both staff and parents at the pool, although (and sadly not uncommonly) no official complaint or report had ever been made to the authorities.

On two occasions, Gerald had followed girls of school age from the swimming pool to their homes and had asked their parents whether in future he could drive the children home in his car; again, no complaint or report was made to the authorities.

On other occasions, Gerald simply followed the children home to find out where they lived. On the next occasion he was at the pool, Gerald would seductively interrogate the children establishing their names, ages or dates of birth, family composition, details of schooling and history. Once in possession of this information, Gerald would send birthday cards and presents to the children, even though he hardly knew them. In addition, he would post Christmas cards to the family, even though he had never met any of the family members.

Gerald skilfully identified a child that most suited his preferences – a pre-teenage junior schoolgirl, who was regularly taken to the swimming pool by a trusted female family friend. The child was supervised by the friend throughout her visit to the pool, but was left alone when making her way home. I shall refer to this child as Janet.

Gerald, having introduced himself, gained the trust of Janet's family friend and engaged in a romantic relationship with her. He was soon introduced to Janet's parents and, after making the offer, was allowed to regularly drive Janet home in his car after the pool sessions had finished. After 12 months the situation had changed dramatically. Gerald had ended his relationship with the family friend, had become a great friend of Janet's and was at this stage allowed to collect her from school, take her to the pool and return her home. Janet's parents also allowed her to venture out with Gerald for daytrips, usually in his campervan, to various places within the UK. On one occasion, Gerald had asked Janet's parents if she could travel with him overnight, but this was refused. Janet was also a regular visitor to Gerald's home and would remain there for several hours at a time.

In addition to establishing a friendship with Janet, Gerald had also imposed himself on Janet's family, becoming a constant and slightly unwelcome visitor to the family home. He began to drive a wedge between Janet and her parents, by providing various gifts such as money, cosmetics and fashionable clothes, as well as transport to wherever she wished to go. These gifts were the sort of things that Janet's parents could not afford or would not allow Janet to have. If Janet wanted to be driven somewhere, or to go into town and her parents refused to take her or would not allow her to go, she would simply call Gerald and he would arrive within minutes and take her wherever she wanted. If Janet and her parents argued, or if Janet did not wish to comply with her parents' requests, she would run from her parents' house and seek sanctuary with Gerald. Gerald would happily allow Janet into his home and let her remain there for as long as she wished.

Initially, Gerald had little to do with Janet or her parents. But as time passed, Janet's parents often found her with quantities of money far in excess of her pocket money allowance. She also had a regular supply of new clothes, shoes, cosmetics, CDs, etc., all given to her by Gerald. Janet's parents had always thought Gerald to be a kind and helpful man and had only disliked his increased calling at the family home. However, by the time of my involvement, Janet's parents were annoyed at Gerald for his continual association with Janet, his giving of gifts and acting as a chauffeur and, more concerning, his ways of undermining their parental control.

Gerald was 'grooming' Janet, by undermining her parents' authority and, by seduction, forming his own pseudo-parental role.

Gerald had always lived with his mother until her death shortly before he began attending the pool. His house was immaculately presented with everything in a well-ordered fashion. Oddly, the house was decorated and furnished in a typical 1950s style. Everything, that is, apart from a new computer with an Internet connection upon which a large number of child/teenage games were installed, a PlayStation, a modern hi-fi and a collection of pop music CDs. These items were not in keeping with the rest of the house, or indeed in keeping with Gerald.

Gerald also possessed a large quantity of photographic equipment and admitted to liking taking photographs of people, particularly Janet.

I formed the opinion that Gerald was a seductive paedophile. Whether he was fixated or regressed (two terms that are explained later in this book) was a matter I would have to discover later. He was sexually attracted towards pre-pubescent girls and had actively engaged in targeting children and parents or carers at the pool. He had found Janet a physically attractive child who was vulnerable, easily manipulated and wishing for far more than her parents could or would allow her. Gerald also found that Janet responded positively to him, when given gifts and favours. He also discovered that Janet's parents and the family friend were all too trusting, too naive and perhaps a little weak-minded.

I spoke to Janet's parents and outlined the common features and behavioural patterns of a paedophile. As I read my notes of Gerald's profile assessment, it was like ticking off a checklist of known and recognisable paedophiliac characteristics.

As you will read in the following pages, paedophiles display a great many typical and identifiable characteristics and behaviours which readily identify them.

Janet's parents could not believe what I was telling them. They felt it impossible that such a pleasant, kind, respectable man, although irritating at times, could possibly act in a sexual manner towards their child. To them he appeared too genuine, too honest, and too normal.

In truth, they did not believe or accept my view. They disregarded the fact that an official had called at their home, highlighting the dangers of this man and listing all his characteristics and behaviours which identified him as a seductive paedophile. As a result, Janet remained at risk.

I was able to immediately disrupt Gerald's activities to a degree by disclosing Gerald's concerning 'attention to children' to the managers of local swimming pools and leisure centres who agreed to refuse him entry should he attend during parent and children's sessions. Local police and other authorities were also informed, and 'child protection procedures' were put into motion.

The issue that greatly concerned me was that I had failed to convince Janet's parents that Gerald posed a threat of significant harm to their daughter. All I had to offer as evidence were a few notes, my explanation of paedophilia from my personal knowledge and experience, and a poorly photocopied leaflet from a children's charity, detailing a few points to consider regarding 'child safety with adults'.

I could not offer Janet's parents anything tangible, any evidence or anything influential in written form. I had nothing in my possession that Janet's parents could mentally ingest, to help them understand and allow them to identify for themselves the risk Gerald posed. I was clearly unable to persuade these parents to appreciate the high-risk situation their daughter was in – a daughter whom I suspected was in the process of being groomed for future sexual abuse.

What I desperately required, in order to convince Janet's parents, that ... MISTER NICE GUY IS ACTUALLY A PAEDOPHILE AND HAS TARGETED YOUR DAUGHTER FOR FUTURE CHILD SEXUAL ABUSE (CSA) ... was an informative, impartial, clear concise guide listing every known characteristic of paedophiles, every known behavioural pattern and grooming method, and every recognisable symptom of child abuse. In other words:

> ... a compilation of information to which parents and carers of children could readily refer and use to identify and recognise the actions and behaviour of paedophiles should a predatory paedophile target their child.

I could find no such guide, so I made the decision to write one.

Adrian Powell
February 2007

About the author

Adrian Powell has worked within the child protection arena since 1997. Primarily, his work has involved sexual risk assessment, monitoring within the community and disruption of paedophiliac and hebephiliac activities, of both registered and non-registered sex offenders and other persons who pose a significant risk of harm to children.

His day-to-day work requires him to interview both perpetrators and victims of child sexual abuse and it is from these interviews and through personal study that the majority of this book's content is derived. In addition, the author has worked alongside many expertly qualified and experienced professionals who work within the numerous child protection agencies, and he has drawn upon their knowledge and skills to assist him in both his vocation and this book.

He maintains his position to this day: promoting child protection awareness and prevention, assessing the risk level presented by known individuals of concern, working to assist in the prosecution of offenders, and monitoring offenders and persons of risk who circulate in our communities.

Acknowledgements

I would like to thank Cheri Powell, Anne Howard and Angela Newman for their encouragement, support and assistance throughout the early stages of this book's development.

Also, I wish to acknowledge all the professionals with whom it has been a privilege to have worked and studied; drawing knowledge and experience from their labour has been of great assistance to me in my vocation within the child protection arena and in the production of this book. Many of these professionals work within agencies and departments of such a kind that it would be inappropriate to list them by name, however they are representative of the Police, Social Services, Local Authority child welfare and education departments, schools, child protection charities and healthcare. Some work alone or for organisations as aids or trainers; people like Ray Wyre CQSW DSW DIP Th [Ray Wyre Associates]; Terry Jones IPTAC, CEOP BA (Hons) PGCE, and Joe Sullivan CEOP MA (Crim) BA (Hons) CQSW Dip Psych, all of whom have devoted years of their lives to protecting children, and constantly strive to help others achieve the same.

Finally, I wish to thank Rachael Redman for her invaluable professional guidance and personal support.

List of abbreviations

CAIT	Child Abuse Investigation Team
CAIU	Child Abuse Investigation Unit
CB	Citizen Band radio
CEOP	Child Exploitation and Online Protection
COPINE	Combating Paedophile Information Networks in Europe
CPAI	Child Physical Abuse Image
CPD	Child Protection Department
CPS	Crown Prosecution Service
CSA	child sexual abuse
CSAI	Child Sexual Abuse Image
EU	European Union
FII	Fabricated and Induced Illness
IIG	Internet Initiated Grooming
IRC	Internet Relay Chat
ISP	Internet Service Provider
IT	information technology
IWF	Internet Watch Foundation
LSCB	Local Safeguarding Children Board
MAPPA	Multi Agency Public Protection Arrangements
NCMEC	National Centre for Missing and Exploited Children
PICS	Platform for Internet Content Selection
POLIT	Paedophile Online Investigation Team
RSACi	Recreational Software Advisory Council
RSHO	Risk of Sexual Harm Order
SOPS	Sexual Offences Prevention Order
SSD	social services department
STD	sexually transmitted disease
UT	urinary tract infection

Introduction

This guide has been produced with one motive:

> To arm protectors of children with the required knowledge and skills to prevent and stop the emotional, physical and sexual abuse of children and child neglect.

Protectors of children – that's you. Whether you are a parent, step-parent, uncle, aunt, grandparent, childminder, child sibling, teacher, health professional, youth worker, foster carer, social worker or an individual totally unconnected with any child, as an adult or as a child, when certain circumstances exist, you can become a protector of children.

There are many aspects of a protector's role which can help to prevent child abuse. While it is clearly idealistic or naive to believe or to suggest that sexual abuse of children can be completely eradicated, it is not beyond possibility that, with appropriate education and guidance, the number of child sexual abuse cases can be greatly reduced. It should be the primary objective of all parents and caring adults to do whatever is possible to stop sexual abuse of children.

I have two main motives in writing this guide. The first is to create and increase awareness among professionals and the public of typical paedophiliac traits and behavioural patterns, sexually motivated grooming techniques, and established facts concerning sexually abusive behaviour inflicted on children. The second is to assist parents and carers in recognising common physical and psychological symptoms of the four main types of child abuse; these are emotional abuse, physical and sexual abuse and neglect.

This guide does not simply 'point out' a few tell-tale signs to '*look out for just in case*'; this guide provides the reader with vital, clear and concise information to assist the reader in detecting abusers and identifying the physical and psychological signs of current and historic child abuse. In addition, this guide sets out relevant information concerning child protection issues and incorporates a working strategy for assessing new friends, professionals or family members as to their suitability to be in contact with children.

Protectors of children can thus identify active, targeting paedophiliac activity, and recognise possible victims. In addition, this guide sets out to dispel the myths and misconceptions about those who sexually abuse children and, where necessary, break down the barriers and prejudices that make people believe 'it will not happen in my family'.

Both sexual assaults and sexually motivated offences against children, including non-contact offences such as 'grooming for sexual acts', are incidences that occur too often, to too many children, in too many families and for too long a

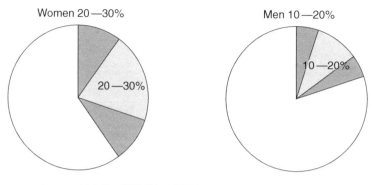

Women 20—30%   Men 10—20%

(sources: Finkelhor 1994; Briere 1990.)

Figure A   20–40% of women and 10–20% of men have been sexually abused as children.

period. It is far more common than most people realise or, as is often the case, are willing to accept.

Studies by Finkelhor (1994) and Briere (1990) suggest that 20–40% women and 10–20% of men have been sexually abused as children (*see* Figure A).

The figures shown will, to any concerned parent or child carer, be shocking and appalling. This evidence should therefore encourage and motivate parents and professionals to gain knowledge and skills to help them protect the children for whom they are responsible.

Detailed and expansive descriptions outlining both the severity of the psychological damage caused by good quality grooming, and a graphic portrayal of the physical harm caused by sexual abuse, would not serve to assist a parent or professional in protecting children. However, I believe that arming parents and professionals with information and skills to help identify the characteristics and behavioural patterns of adults with a sexual interest in children definitely will.

I do not profess however that every characteristic, every behavioural pattern and every grooming method is detailed within the following pages. Nevertheless, I do profess to having collated a great number of such characteristics and behavioural patterns and outlined them in such a fashion as to be easily understood and recognisable. I do not claim to be an expert, or allege to be profoundly qualified in the area of 'sexual abuser assessment or treatment', but I have studied sexually abusive behaviour for many years and write with a combination of knowledge gained predominantly from my own practical experience and the work of other practitioners.

I must stress that, in my attempt to explain how and why some people sexually abuse children, I do not in any way condone or excuse their behaviour.

Generalisations

This guide is aimed at all persons who care for and have responsibility for children, including parents and guardians of children as well as professionals working in the field of child protection such as health professionals, social service professionals, education welfare officers, teachers, childcare staff, police officers, and accident and emergency hospital staff. Throughout this guide parents and guardians will be referred to as 'carers', and persons employed with child protection responsibility will be referred to as 'professionals'.

Each section is divided into 'bite-sized' chapters. Four particular areas of child protection are described which will greatly assist parents and professionals in identifying potential or active abusers. The guide will also assist in the identification, prevention and ending of current abuse. The abuse types outlined in the section on the signs and symptoms of abuse are emotional, physical and sexual abuse and neglect.

When a sexual offender's characteristics and behavioural patterns are identified and acted upon correctly, child abuse and/or further child abuse can be prevented. Such correct action by a parent or professional may also assist in the apprehension of the abuser or abusers.

What is the purpose of each section?

Section One: Identifying paedophiles through behaviour

1   To provide a clear, concise and a no-nonsense approach to the recognition and identification of adults and young persons who possess a sexual interest in children, by outlining their characteristics, practices and behavioural patterns. This will enable the parent or professional to identify a sexual abuser of children should they have the misfortune to encounter such an individual who has targeted their child for future sexual abuse and is attempting to infiltrate their family.
2   To promote a responsible reaction, and clearly detail an individual's duty having detected a sexual abuser or sexual abuse activity.
3   To promote a responsible reaction, and clearly detail an individual's duty when suspecting a person of sexual abuse activity.

Section Two: Recognising symptoms of child abuse

1   To help parents and guardians understand that the 'unbelievable' and the 'unimaginable' does happen.
2   To enable every parent, carer, health and education professional to easily recognise the 'not always' so obvious symptoms of emotional, physical or sexual abuse or neglect displayed by children.
3   To arm relatives, friends and those who work with children with the relevant knowledge to identify symptoms of child abuse, should the abuse come from within the child's family group.
4   To provide a common-sense approach for parents and guardians to protect their children and others' children.

Section Three: The Internet – dangers and safeguards

1   To inform parents and carers of children of how easily a child can become exposed to a targeting child sex abuser while innocently utilising the Internet. Also to outline important information concerning the Internet from a parental or carer's perspective.

2 To show by detailed description how child sex abusers utilise the Internet in both illegal and immoral ways, focusing on targeting, grooming and entrapment.

Section Four: Action – by you and by others

1 To present a method which assists parents and carers of children in recognising and recording the activities that expose sexual abusers of children.
2 To outline actions and best practice that should be considered by parents, child carers and other professionals when first receiving disclosure of child sexual abuse.
3 To detail an overview of police and social services procedures.
4 To put forward an overview of the Sex Offenders Act 1997, the Sexual Offences Act 2000, the Criminal Justice and Court Services Act 2000 and the Sexual Offences Act 2003.

Terminology

To generalise in any field of work can be dangerous and misleading, sometimes with severe consequences. When working in the arena of child protection, it is exceptionally important to use accurate and correct terminology.

For example, I prefer the term 'adults with a sexual interest in children' to that of 'paedophile'. In Chapter 1, 'Understanding sexual orientation and paedophilia', the specifics of paedophilia, hebephilia, ephebophilia and pederast and others are explained. For the purposes of simplicity, I use the term 'paedophile' throughout my guide, but thought must be given to the fact that paedophilia is only one area of child sexual and emotional attraction and a number of adults qualifying for other named terms or labels are equally sexually and emotionally attracted to children.

Throughout this guide, reference is made to specific paedophile activity and behaviour. True personal details are obviously not recorded, but the events are real, as are the feelings and beliefs of the offenders.

Based upon findings by psychologists, other medical practitioners, law courts and the Home Office it is widely recognised that paedophilia exists in men and women, though it is also well documented that the vast majority of paedophiles, both fixated and regressed, are men. It is also recognised, by the same officialdom, that a greater number of girls than boys are sexually abused.

To prevent having to repeatedly describe the *'paedophile'* as *he* or *she*, the guide is written as if the paedophile is always male. It must be accepted that in many of the following described situations, scenarios and references, the paedophile could easily be *male* or *female*. In the same light, irrespective of the type of abuse being described, the victim, in this guide, will always be referred to as *female* unless a specific is required.

References

Briere J, editor. *Assessing and Treating Victims of Violence*. San Francisco: Jossey-Bass; 1990.
Finkelhor D 1994. www.nycagainstrape.org/research_factsheet_7.html

Child abusers – who are they?

Most people have a preconceived notion as to the image and demeanour of a sexual abuser of children. However, in the vast majority of cases, these perceptions will be wrong, and it is important to recognise that having such fundamentally inaccurate ideas can lead to disastrous consequences.

If parents and professionals have a wrong conception concerning the description and behaviour of a sexual abuser, then they are likely to pass the same conception to the children they care for. For example, if someone believes that a child molester is commonly an ugly, horrible-looking, gruff monster of a man who is also smelly, dirty and scruffy, who wears a shabby raincoat and spends most of the time loitering about schools or public toilets, then they may well influence the child for whom they are providing care that 'molesters of children' really are ugly, horrible-looking, gruff monsters of men who are also smelly, dirty and scruffy, wear shabby raincoats and loiter about schools and toilets. Consequently, if a child is approached by a sexual abuser whose appearance is 'normal' and who is clean and well presented and appears to the child to be friendly and attentive, the child is unlikely to think that such a man may pose a real and significant threat.

It must also be remembered that, for a child, a stranger may only be a stranger for a few seconds, particularly if the stranger is skilled at communicating with children and acts in a friendly manner.

Sexual abusers are rarely scruffy, dirty old men wearing greasy raincoats and thick-rimmed glasses who loiter about children's play areas, public toilets or schools, offering children sweets and an opportunity to see their puppies. The vast majority of sexual abusers look normal – they represent a heterogeneous group of individuals. Skilled, determined and experienced, sexual abusers blend into our society and are rarely identified by their appearance. In fact, the most successful sexual abusers work hard not to draw undue attention to themselves by dressing exactly as anyone else would in any given environment or situation. Most sexual abusers also remain unobtrusive by behaving normally and adopting a socially acceptable attitude. Towards other adults they are usually quiet natured, often non-confrontational and conciliatory.

Anyone you know could be an abuser, either sexually, emotionally, physically or by way of neglect. The sexual abuser can be a family member, a family friend, member of the clergy, adoptive parents, a neighbour, a youth worker, teacher, doctor, the over-helpful new partner in your life or the retired quiet gentleman residing at the end of the street. Many sexual abusers of children study or work to achieve positions of trust or employment in areas where children are often the focal point.

It is worthy of note that there are certain occupational groups and types of organisations still in existence today which protect their offending members by simply relocating them rather than reporting the abuse to the authorities.

What is surprising to a great many people is that the sexual abuser can also be another child. Research has shown that 40% of sexual abuse of children can be attributed to older siblings (NSPCC Full-Stop Campaign 2000).

The children's charity ChildLine produces an Annual Review containing statistics regarding abusers. The statistics are based on information gleaned from the children and young people who call ChildLine. The Review gives a breakdown of how many sexual abusers are known or not known to the victim, and, if known, whether they are family or friends (ChildLine Annual Review 2005).

The 2001 Annual Review revealed that in 58% of the cases of sexual abuse reported by children or young people, the abuser was a member of their family. In 32% of the cases the abuser was known to the caller, but not a family member. Only 10% of callers said that they were being sexually abused by a person or persons unknown to them (*see* Figure B).

ChildLine's Annual Review for the year 2005 shows a slight change in the percentage figures, but the over-riding fact remains that intrafamilial sexual abuse is the most common.

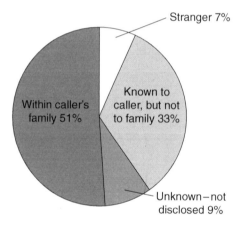

(source: Childline Annual Review 2005)

Figure B   Breakdown (in percentage) of victim's familiarity with the abuser.

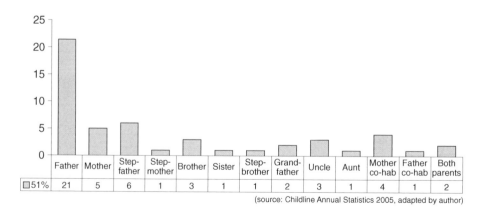

(source: Childline Annual Statistics 2005, adapted by author)

Figure C   Breakdown (in percentage) of intrafamilial abuse.

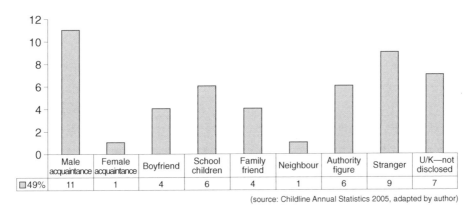

	Male acquaintance	Female acquaintance	Boyfriend	School children	Family friend	Neighbour	Authority figure	Stranger	U/K—not disclosed
☐ 49%	11	1	4	6	4	1	6	9	7

(source: Childline Annual Statistics 2005, adapted by author)

Figure D   Breakdown (in percentage) of non-intrafamilial abuse.

ChildLine's statistics for 2005, obtained from children and young people who called them, demonstrate the breakdown of sexually abusive family members, persons known and persons unknown to the victim (*see* Figure C).
National statistics show that:

- approximately 70% of sexual abusers of children are known to their victims with approximately 80% of the offences taking place in either the offender's or victim's home
- 60–70% of sexual abusers of children target only girls
- 20–33% target boys
- 10% target either sex.

Fisher (1994) stated (making reference to Wolf 1984) that:

... it is a general finding of surveys of sex offender populations that variables such as level of intelligence, age, ethnicity, education and psychiatric status do not differ significantly from the rates in the general populations from which the samples are drawn.

Abusers transcend all classes – they can hold high office and appear as pillars of society; conversely they may be community vagabonds. Sexual abusers can be found in every race, in every culture, in most religions and in any country.
Statistics also show that adult males carry out the vast majority of sexual offences against children, with adult females committing approximately 5% of such offences. In the majority of offences committed by female paedophiles, the victims are the abuser's own children. There is no evidence that adult female paedophiles abuse children of one gender more than the other.
Children and adolescents are also known to sexually abuse other children and other adolescents. Approximately 30% of sexual abusers of children are themselves teenagers. A worrying feature of those who commit child sexual abuse offences is that, unlike any other form of crime, the rate and severity of offending (or the wish to offend) is very likely to increase as the offender ages. The rate of re-offending is also of major concern as it is estimated that a paedophiliac abuser is 90% likely to re-offend; alarmingly only 20% of paedophiles

convicted for sexual abuse of a child are likely to be convicted again for a similar offence. For some paedophiles, however, committing sexual offences may not be frequent; decades can separate one set of offences from another. This is often the case if the offending paedophile has never been caught and convicted, and subsequently forced to undergo a structured Sex Offender Treatment Program.

Both the prison service and the probation service have studied sex offending recidivism and have established that paedophiles who are not related to the children they sexually abuse pose a far greater risk of re-offending.

References

ChildLine. *Annual Review 2005 – perpetrators of sexual abuse*. 2005. www.childline.org. uk/Annualreview.asp

Fisher L 1994. www.nspcc.org.uk/Inform/OnlineResources/InformationBriefings/ASO_ asp_ifega26012.html

NSPCC. *Full-Stop Campaign*. 2000. www.nspcc.org.uk

Wolf 1984. www.nspcc.org.uk/Inform/OnlineResources/InformationBriefings/ASO_ asp_ifega26012.html

How to use this guide

- Study this guide, and other suggested information sources (*see* Appendix B), in order to develop an understanding of paedophilia and hebephilia.
- Be aware of the typical history, lifestyle and common circumstances in which paedophiles and hebephiles involuntarily exist.
- Learn to identify the often-shielded typical behavioural characteristics that active predatory paedophiles and hebephiles display.
- From then on, use this guide as a reference tool whenever you or your child is befriended by, or introduced to, a 'new' person (*see* Section Four).
- Remember, paedophiles and hebephiles can be male or female (in this guide, they are always referred to as males).
- Familiarise yourself with often overlooked signs and symptoms of active abuse displayed by a child. Be aware that they can be the result of any one of the four main abuse types or a combination.
- Develop an understanding with your child concerning all aspects of abuse. Break down the barriers that may exist which prevent your child talking with you or to others about child abuse.
- Most offending paedophiles re-offend. Understand the cycle of offending so as to accept and recognise how they justify their behaviour to themselves, distort their thinking, fantasise, and motivate themselves into offending.
- Be aware of what lies ahead for you and your child once a referral has been made to the police or social services.
- Become familiar with the law pertaining to sexual offending, registered sex offenders and the various prohibitive orders that can be imposed upon offenders.
- Finally, consider using the checklists in Section Four to record characteristics and behaviour displayed by a potentially abusive person.

Section One

Identifying paedophiles through behaviour

Understanding sexual orientation and paedophilia

What is sexual orientation?

By definition it is:

Sexual   *adj*   pertaining to sex or the sexes; having sex.
Orientation   *n*   arrangement; alignment; one's way of thinking; one's direction of interest.

Sexual orientation is psychological. It is one's preference of the gender, age range and physical appearance of another, to which one is emotionally attracted and sexually aroused.

In short; it is one's mental view of the 'sexual ideal'.

Heterosexual   sexually orientated to persons of the opposite sex (or gender).
Homosexual   sexually orientated to persons of the same sex (or gender).

The majority of human beings are born with a single pre-determined gender-specific sexual orientation, and possess within the orientation preferences such as age, build, hair colour, eye colour, etc. Others are born with both sexual orientations and again possess particular preferences. Such people will generally experience having one dominant orientation. However, for those individuals possessing multi-orientations, illness, disabilities, social factors, poor education, a limited choice of available sexual partners, or any number of circumstances may cause an individual's true sexual orientation to be subdued or even prevented from developing. Suppression of true sexual feelings or urges is very common and, on occasions, it is not until later in life that an individual may have the courage, strength or ability to engage in the type of sexual and emotional relationship they crave.

In the United Kingdom the only sexual orientations deemed socially and legally acceptable are:

adult male (16 years +)   with   adult female (16 years +)
adult male (16 years +)   with   adult male (16 years +)
adult female (16 years +)   with   adult female (16 years +)

United Kingdom law allows people to have sexual intercourse with willing participants over the age of 16.

It is illegal for anyone to have sexual intercourse with someone under the age of 16 years. In today's society, it is unacceptable for anyone, adult or child, to have a sexual orientation towards children.

What must be understood is that where an adult male may be sexually aroused by an adult female due to her looks, her voice, her walk, and her dress code, etc., another adult may experience the exact same emotions and arousal by the sight, sound, movement and dress code, etc., of a child.

Most non-paedophiliac members of society consider people who are aroused by children as being 'sick', 'deranged', 'mental' or 'subnormal'. Some are and some are not.

But what if ...

Consider what it must be like if, for genetic reasons, you pass through childhood and adolescence, and enter into adulthood having never experienced sexual arousal by adult females or males. You are in a world where sexual desire, sexual arousal and sexual gratification can only be achieved with the involvement of children. For some, this would be a living hell from which they strive to escape. For others, this is a natural behaviour, believing that sexually fantasising about children, and engaging in sexual activity with children, is not wrong.

Paedophilia and hebephilia

For generations, society has used the term 'paedophile' to define, in most cases, 'an adult who possesses an unnatural, sexual attraction towards children', where the age or physical development of the child is not defined. Therefore, society generally accepts the term paedophile to mean an adult who is sexually attracted to a child of any age or sexual maturity. However, those identified as having a sexual interest in children can be divided into two main groups depending on the age and sexual maturity of the children to whom they are attracted. These groups are paedophiles and hebephiles.

What is a paedophile?

By definition a paedophile is:

> **Paedophile** *adj* a person with a sexual desire directed towards children.

True meanings

> **'Phile'** A Greek term deriving from the word 'philia', said to describe 'love' or 'deep friendship'.

Paedophile

Etymological meaning: *Pede-* or *Paedo-* is derived from the Greek word 'Paido', which means 'boy' or 'child'. The word *'Paidophiles'* appears to refer, in ancient times, to an adult male who fell in love with, and became sexually involved with, boys.

Clinical meaning: An adult (male or female) who is emotionally and/or sexually attracted to pre-pubescent children.

Lay meaning: An adult (male or female) who is attracted to pre-pubescent children; an adult who molests children; a child who is attracted to, or molests younger children (very often within the family).

Heterosexual paedophiles

Persons with a sexual and erotic preference for children of the opposite sex who fall within an average age range up to and including 11 or 12 years of age; in any case, children who do not physically display sexual maturity (pre-pubescent).

Homosexual paedophiles

Persons with a sexual and erotic preference for children of the same sex who fall within an average age range up to and including 11 or 12 years of age; in any case, children who do not physically display sexual maturity (pre-pubescent).

What is a hebephile?

By definition a hebephile is:

Hebephile

Etymological meaning: the Liddell-Scott 'Greek–English Lexicon' describes the term *hebe* as 'the time before manhood, at Athens 16 years of age'. Other references read 'the time before 14' and 'the time before 18'. Generally, the term *hebe* is taken from the Greek deity Hebe, the goddess and protectoress of adolescents – referred to in Greek culture as 'youth'.

Clinical meaning: An adult who is sexually and emotionally attracted to adolescents (younger than 18).

Lay meaning: It is not common to find this word being used in everyday speech.

Heterosexual hebephile

Persons with a sexual and erotic preference for pubescent young people of the opposite sex, commonly aged 11 to 14 for girls, and 15 or 16 for boys.

Homosexual hebephile

Persons with a sexual and erotic preference for pubescent young people of the same sex, commonly aged 11 to 14 for girls, and 15 or 16 for boys.

> **Note**
> An offender's sexual orientation, whether he perceives himself as homosexual, heterosexual or bisexual, is not considered as a risk factor, indicator or characteristic in typologies of child sex offenders. (Finkelhor, Williams, Burns and Kalinowski 1988)

Most paedophiles and hebephiles are male and most will target female victims.

In the vast majority of known cases, paedophiles and hebephiles are males who are drawn towards female children. However, this is not always the case. An adult's heterosexuality or homosexuality is not an indication as to the abuser's sexual preference of children.

As an example, an adult male abuser may prefer to sexually abuse male children aged between six years and eight years while maintaining a heterosexual relationship with an adult female.

It is important to remember that paedophilia and hebephilia does not exist solely among males. Although only a small number, a proportion of adult women have a sexual orientation towards children; such women invariably sexually abuse their own children.

Lesser-known terms

Chronophile

Chronophiles are persons of any age whose sexuoerotic age is incongruous with their physical age, yet is harmonious with the age of their chosen sexual partner/preference. Chronophilia is not related in any way to paedophilia, hebephilia, ephebophilia, gerontophilia or teleiophilia as individuals who possess these sexual orientations have congruent physical and sexuoerotic ages and generally have a preference for people of a different physical age.

Ephebophile

The Liddell-Scott 'Greek–English Lexicon' describes the term ephebos as meaning 'one arrived at adolescence'. The term was also used to describe 'young boy' and/or 'young girl'. In principle, the term means: an adult who is sexually and emotionally attracted to adolescents; an adult who is attracted to adolescents younger than 18.

Gerontophile

A gerontophile is a person, male or female, who is sexually attracted to, or has a sexual preference for, people significantly older than themselves. In general terms: a gerontophile is a young or non-elderly individual, who possesses a sexual attraction or a sexual preference towards elderly people.

Teleiophile

A teleiophile is a child or an adolescent who is sexually attracted to adults.
(Further information relating to the vulnerability of gerontophiles and teleiophiles is outlined in Chapter 3.)

Paraphile

A term often used to describe one of a number of sexual preferences in which an adult's sexual arousal or sexual fantasy consists of sexual activity involving non-human objects, children or adolescents, other non-consenting individuals, or the infliction of pain upon another.

Pederast

Also known as the Shotaro Complex. Similarly to the word paedophile, pederast is derived from the Greek word paidos, which means 'boy' or 'child'. Pederast was a synonym for paedophile, referring to a male adult who experiences emotional and sexual desire for, and engages in penetrative anal sex with, male adolescents. The term also refers to adult women who are sexually and emotionally attracted to adolescent boys or girls.

Lolita

Also known as the Lolita Complex. Often used to refer to adults or children, attracted to adolescent or older underage *female*s.

Nepiophilia

Also called infantophilia. This term describes adults who are sexually attracted to 'babies' or 'infants'. The age of preference can range between nought and three years. Research has been conducted which suggests a distinction between paedophilia and nepiophilia, as it is believed that paedophilies are rarely sexually aroused by babies or infants.

The intention of both professionals and the public to use the correct terminology when describing adults who are sexually attracted to children is good, but fraught with danger. Such good intentions can easily be misinterpreted as the terminology used is often imprecise, unfamiliar and far too general. Throughout this guide, for simplicity and clarity, I refer to people who are sexually attracted to children of any age or physical development as paedophiles.

Paedophilia is a mental state whereby the individual is sexually aroused by the sight, sounds or smells of a child. For a paedophile, the desire for sex with a child is equally as strong as a heterosexual adult desiring sex with an adult member of the opposite sex or a homosexual desiring sex with an adult person of his or her own gender. Paedophilia is not an illness. It is not a passing phase. Although recognised as not being an illness but a generic sexual orientation, having paedophiliac tendencies is not an excuse for offending. There is no cure – only control, most of which must be generated by the paedophile himself. Even the highly involved 'Sex Offender Treatment Programmes' initiated and maintained by the Prison Service and Probation Service cannot guarantee that a high- or low-risk sex offender will not re-offend.

It must be accepted and understood that not all paedophiles are male. There are female paedophiles, but far fewer of them. As with male paedophiles, their paedophilia will be heterosexual, homosexual or a combination.

Paedophiles may appear perfectly respectable, plausible and genuinely nice people. They may not look like 'dirty old men' or society's stereotypical 'pervert'. Paedophiles can be found in every walk of life, every race and any form of religion. They are classless; they can exist as pillars of the community and as down-and-outs. Respectable uncles, loving granddads and favourite aunts can all fit the bill.

Paedophiles have definite characteristics that can be clearly identified; they can be *predatory* and therefore be a major threat to the welfare of children. Paedophiles are often found to be extremely intelligent people, able to gain the confidence of their proposed victim and the proposed victim's family. Others are passive and can pose little threat to children, focusing on fantasy and masturbation.

Once a paedophile chooses to sexually offend against a child, the offending and preparation for offending becomes compulsive; it is not a 'one-off' act. It is ongoing behaviour that involves the corruption of a relationship over a period of time. The abuser will select a 'safe' victim and will continue offending against that victim until such time as the victim no longer falls within the abuser's preferred age range or preferred sexual maturity.

Paedophiles fall into one of two categories:

1 fixated paedophile
2 regressed paedophile.

(*See* Chapter 2, 'Two types of paedophile and their typical characteristics'.)

Within each of these defined groups are further descriptive categories.

Offending paedophiles, either fixated or regressed, will be described by some as *predatory*. Other offending paedophiles, again either fixated or regressed, will be described as *seductive*. I believe that these descriptive categories are sometimes inappropriate, as they tend to suggest that paedophiles are either one or the other. I consider that paedophiles are capable of being one or both.

As examples:

A paedophile abducting a child and subjecting the child to immediate sexual abuse could easily be described as predatory. He has acted either with the intent to abduct and abuse or has been presented with an unforeseen opportunity to abduct and abuse, as a predator – by being prepared to sexually abuse a child, striking at random.

A paedophile that proactively searches for a child to abuse, identifies a potential victim and conducts a number of planned actions to befriend, seduce and abuse the child could also be considered predatory as well as seductive. He displays a predatory nature by virtue of his searching and targeting of potential victims. However, his approach is seductive and would be considered by the paedophile as 'relationship building'.

A paedophile that has about him, or within easy access, potential victims may well only be seductive. A good example of a purely seductive paedophile would be a grandfather who abuses, for the first time in his life, his regularly visiting grandchildren.

Explanations of the types of paedophile are detailed in later chapters; their categories that fall within the headings of fixated, regressed, predatory or seductive are clearly definable. These categories can be titled as: homosexual, heterosexual, bisexual, sadistic, masochistic, voyeuristic – in fact any sexual orientation or perversion usually associated with an adult's relationship with another adult can be found to exist in a relationship between the paedophile and his victim.

We must realise, however, that not every paedophile will physically abuse a child.

Not all paedophiles offend against children. Some are able to control their fantasies, urges and desires and will never harm a child. Such paedophiles are still aroused by children and may well fantasise about children but will utilise photographic material, written material or adults role-playing as children to satisfy their sexual needs.

We must also realise that some paedophiles, being highly intelligent, predatory, well-organised, learned, plausible, good communicators, dedicated to their goal, remorseless, manipulative, ruthless and, in some cases, deadly, pose the highest risk of harm possible to society's children.

We must also remember that a child can be sexually abused by another child. This is more likely to be an act of experimentation or a misunderstanding of adult issues, witnessed by the child possibly from television or other adults. However, as an example, a 12-year-old boy can be fully aware of what he is doing to a nine-year-old girl.

Reference

Finkelhor D, Williams LM, Burns N, Kalinowski M. *Sexual Abuse in Day Care: a national study. Executive summary*. Durham, NH: Family Research Laboratory; 1998. Quoted in: www.aifs.gov.au/nch/issues5.html.

Two types of paedophile and their typical characteristics

Characteristics of the regressed paedophile

By definition:

Regressed *adj* to fall back, retire, relapse or degenerate.

An example of a regressed paedophile's typical circumstances and activity

The offender, an adult male, marries an adult female. They have children who grow into adults and have children of their own. The offender and the offender's wife throughout this period have maintained a healthy heterosexual relationship. As time passes and the offender and his wife reach their sixties and seventies, the offender's wife becomes less interested in sexual activity. The offender maintains his sexual urges and desires, and seeks sexual activity with an adult female. Due, possibly, to his increasing age and changing physical appearance, he is unable to establish a relationship with a female of his true sexual desire.

He becomes desperate for any form of arousal and sexual activity. In his desperation, he accepts that he must obtain sexual gratification from whatever source is available. The availability of a sexual source is crucial but, unfortunately for him, such sources are rare. However, his grandchildren are available to him and trust him, as do his own children. The abuse can begin with inappropriate tickling and play fighting. This can develop into minor indecent assaults that are usually considered by the victim to be either accidental inappropriate touching, or acceptable deliberate touching, as the child victim has no notion that the behaviour is wrong. Eventually, through seduction or control, the abuse can develop into acts of horrific indecent assault or even rape.

In these circumstances, it is not definite that the offender is a true paedophile; he may be deriving physical sexual gratification from the child, but is at the same time probably fantasising about his ideal adult female.

'Not every sex offender against a child is a true paedophile, sometimes the child serves only as a substitute for a mature partner.' A study by Hall *et al.* of Kent State University, for example, found that 32.5% of their sample – consisting of eighty adult males – exhibited sexual arousal to heterosexual paedophilic stimuli that equalled or exceeded their arousal to the adult stimuli. Further studies indicate that even men erotically fixated on adult females are generally prone to react sexually when exposed to nude female children. (Freund 1990).

The offender may have control of his victim or victims through fear. He may be telling his victim or victims that they will be taken from their parents if they tell anyone about what's going on. Or he may be telling them that 'all granddads do this' and that 'it is just our little secret'.

Some offenders, who have pleaded guilty to such crimes committed in these circumstances, claim that their plea was to prevent the child having to suffer further strain and upset by having to attend court. In doing so, many offenders convince themselves that they have 'done their victims a favour' and that the said victims 'owe' the offenders a favour in return.

Regressed paedophiles will display one or more of the following characteristics

Primary sexual arousal and orientation, originally directed towards adults, becomes directed towards children

As an adolescent and as an adult, the regressed paedophile's sexual arousal and orientation has been drawn towards adults.

This is true whether the regressed paedophile is heterosexual or homosexual. In other words, the regressed paedophile, through puberty and through at least part of his adult life, is sexually stimulated by the sight and sounds, etc., of adults. Having reached adulthood, young or old, the regressed paedophile will at some time in the future begin to find an interest, a fascination, sexual arousal and desire for children.

Initially, focusing on children will be impulsive

The regressed paedophile is unlikely to have a well-structured, developed and organised method of offending, though this may well change with experience. He will act in a rash and hasty fashion, offending when the opportunity arises and under the sway of his emotions.

Stress is a common precipitating factor

Mental stress can affect everyone and can affect its sufferers in various ways.

When a regressed paedophile has his life in control and life in general is pleasing (sexual relationship with adult partner is adequate, has a good lifestyle, is respected by peers, holds down a decent job, etc. – all that causes little or no stress), it is unlikely that he will allow his desire for children to increase at that time. If, however, the regressed paedophile, who recognises his sexual persuasion as being paedophiliac or hebephiliac, experiences high levels of stress in his life, he may well have his interests and desires for sexual involvement with a child heightened and extenuated.

The regressed paedophile will usually be married or be in a common-law relationship. He may well be a parent and abandon his parental role. The victim is seen as a pseudo-adult

A regressed paedophile may spend many years as an adult enjoying sexual activity with other adults either in marriage or common-law relationships. He may be a parent or at least understand parental roles and responsibilities. He will ignore this parental role and carry no feeling of responsibility for, or accountability towards, a child. He may have lost the availability of a sexually active adult partner and may find that, for whatever reason, he can only establish relationships with children. It is possible in these circumstances for the regressed paedophile to fantasise that the child he is abusing is an adult.

Most paedophiles are male and most will target female victims

In the vast majority of known cases, regressed paedophiles are males who are drawn towards female children. However, this is not always the case. An adult's heterosexuality or homosexuality is not an indication as to the abuser's sexual preference of children.

As an example, an adult male abuser may prefer to sexually abuse male children aged between six years and eight years while maintaining a heterosexual relationship with an adult female.

The use of alcohol is often related to the act

A regressed paedophile may be at a stage where he is on the verge of offending. He is prevented from doing so by his own self-control (internal inhibitors), because of the fear of retribution, of being caught and the ensuing prosecution, or because of genuine concern for the child victim.

Alcohol can disable an individual's self-control, increasing disinhibitors and causing an otherwise rational and level-headed person to act without sense or reason.

Some regressed paedophiles may purposefully consume alcohol to both boost their confidence in offending and assist with reducing or eliminating their internal inhibitors; others may innocently consume alcohol and unwittingly achieve the same state of mind.

Possible reasons for regression

Paedophiliac regression may occur due to one or more of the following being an element in a man's life, and may lead to sexual offending: poor quality lifestyle, little sense of direction, feelings of hopelessness, underdeveloped peer relationships, isolation in his own mind, continual failure in his exploits, becoming physically unattractive to adult women either due to age, illness or accident.

It must be understood that many men and women experience one or more of the above, but do not develop a sexual interest in children. All of these elements, however, bring with them a level of stress – stress which may cause a few somewhat sexually normative adults to focus sexually on a child.

Characteristics of the fixated paedophile

By definition:

> **Fixated**   *adj*   to make stable, establish, definite, decided, to set in order, set to remain permanently.

Involuntary (personal) characteristics and behaviour

Primary sexual orientation and arousal is directed towards children

Throughout adolescence and adulthood (and, in many cases, throughout early childhood) the fixated paedophile has experienced sexual arousal when watching or fantasising about children, and has desired sexual activity with children. The fixated paedophile's orientation is psychological and deep rooted. It is as normal to him as desiring members of the opposite sex is to heterosexuals and desiring the same sex is to homosexuals.

Paedophilia is not an illness; it is an incurable mental state.

Illegal paedophiliac behaviour can only be prevented with the use of control – either by the paedophile's self-control (internal inhibitors) or by society, i.e. prison, monitoring within the community or sex offender treatment programmes (external inhibitors).

It must be remembered that not all paedophiles physically offend. Some use other means of obtaining sexual gratification, such as the illegal viewing of indecent images of children while masturbating, or having consenting adults role-play as children during sexual activity.

Interest begins during adolescence

As paedophilia is not an illness but a generic sexual orientation, it is present throughout the paedophile's life. When a young male or female passes through puberty, he or she will develop both physically and psychologically. Psychologically, males and females develop an interest in the adult characteristics of members of the same or opposite sex. Paedophiles will, of course, develop an interest in other children. Pubescent and pre-pubescent children will have a desire to 'play' with the genitals of other children – in many cases, this is a cousin or younger sibling. Their sexual interest in pubescent and/or pre-pubescent children does not diminish and is carried with them throughout their lives.

Some adults, during therapeutic treatment, have stated that their sexual interest in pubescent or pre-pubescent children began early in their lives, some as young as seven years of age.

Has strong cognitive distortions

Many offenders of paedophiliac crimes express having certain 'beliefs', which they draw upon to account for their offending.

They include:

'That is what children are on the earth for.'
'I was sexually abused as a child, so I'll do it to others.'

'It's been going on for thousands of years, so what's the problem?'
'It feels natural to me; I love children and would not cause them any lasting harm.'
'My wife and I don't have sex, so having sex with my daughter keeps the family together' and
'What I did was very minimal in the grand scale of things. I only touched her; I didn't do anything serious.'

Some offenders genuinely believe that what they do is not wrong and their actions are normal and acceptable to others.

May be well ordered and precise

The majority of paedophiles are known to have a tendency of being very well organised, meticulous and precise about all their activities. They appear to like possessions, documents, videos, etc., to be clearly marked or labelled, stacked or placed in a form of recognised order. They will keep meticulous records of activities and meetings. Everything must be neat and tidy. The majority of paedophiles also maintain a high standard of personal hygiene and present themselves, if not well dressed, then smartly dressed.

Fails to develop good peer-group relationships

The majority of paedophiles do not interact successfully with peer adult groups of either gender. They fail to enjoy good relationships with men or women of equal intellectual or social standing. They are usually loners and, if they do have friends, these friends and friendships are likely to be business-like with other paedophiles. As paedophiles are usually lonely characters and are unable to share their interests, ideals, plans and successes with many others, any information gleaned regarding victims or possible victims is very likely to be shared with paedophiliac associates. Such associations are usually born out of enforced contact in prison or during therapeutic group work; some are generated through Internet websites or chat rooms.

Will claim offence was 'totally out of character' and a 'one-off' occurrence

Unless confronted with evidence showing a catalogue of offences, the paedophile will claim his actions were either unforeseen, due to stress, a misunderstanding, drug or alcohol related. Anything, except the truth.

Voluntary (personally chosen) circumstances and behaviour of the fixated paedophile

Usually lives alone or with his mother, sometimes with both parents

A good number of paedophiles are 'loners' and live alone. This is mainly due to their inability to develop good and proper relationships with peers. Living alone also increases security about their activities and the secrecy of their desires. Many paedophiles, again due to poor relationships with peers, remain with their parents until their parents' death. This also provides security and safety as many parents refuse to accept that their offspring could ever be an offending paedophile.

Rarely will a fixated paedophile marry. If he does so or enters into a common-law relationship, it will very likely be a marriage or relationship of 'convenience'

If a fixated paedophile marries or engages in a common-law relationship, he is either:

- In full control of his emotions and sexual desires towards children and can suppress the urges typical of a paedophile by strong mental will and utilising alternative sexual activity. His partner may be fully aware of his preferences and engage in child role-play by performing sex acts dressed as and/or acting as a child.
- Marrying to portray a 'normal' heterosexual relationship in an attempt to distract attention or suspicion of being a paedophile. This will often help the paedophile gain the trust of other adults who see him as a happily married person and therefore unlikely to have a sexual interest in children. He may become a parent within this relationship and will possibly be of no threat to his own offspring.
- Entering into marriage or, more likely, a common-law relationship with a single parent to gain access to children. Depending upon the age of the paedophile, the children concerned may be the new partner's children, grandchildren, nieces or nephews or even children to whom the new partner has access/contact, e.g. the new partner is a youth club worker, teacher, childcarer/babysitter.

If he has friends, they are usually also paedophiles

Due to their secret behaviour, illegal material kept at home and their wishes to maintain a low profile, paedophiles are generally loners. They will not set out to meet, socialise and genuinely befriend people who are not paedophiles themselves. They will only befriend other paedophiles or people who present an opportunity for them to gain access to children.

Will circulate information regarding possible/suitable victims with other paedophiles

To maintain a high level of activity and regular sexual activity with children, many paedophiles liaise with other paedophiles either individually or as organised groups. The following is a list outlining the type of information paedophiles will share with other paedophiles:

- details of current and past victims
- access routes to vulnerable children and victims
- locations of vulnerable children and possible victims such as special schools, clubs, hostels, associations, etc.

- methods and tips on grooming
- suppliers of videos and magazines containing indecent images of children
- Internet sites of interest to paedophiles
- the identities of paedophiles engaged in organised sexual abuse of children (child sex rings).

As an example, if a 'supply' of vulnerable children is identified by a paedophile (say a group of children housed by the local authority who disregard the authority's rules thereby endangering themselves by being open to paedophiliac seduction) he may inform other paedophiles of this group. He will hope that all the children will be 'controlled' by a number of paedophiles so that he can conduct sexual activities with one or more of the children at any one time. By introducing other paedophiles, he is also encouraging other paedophiles to introduce him to other vulnerable children in the future.

Utilises material that is either 'indecently child-erotic' or 'lawful' but found to be child-erotic by the paedophile

Whether a paedophile is actively offending or not, he is very likely to make use of child-erotic material.

The term 'child-erotic material' is not a term that I consider appropriate. Like the term 'child pornography' it tends to suggest that the children involved are willing participants, fully aware and consenting to being photographed or filmed, much like the adult 'porn' star. This material is better described as 'material containing indecent images of children' or 'abusive images'.

The material concerned will contain either images solely of children, children interacting sexually with other children or adults, or children interacting sexually with animals. Conversely, the material may contain images combining variants of all three. The collected material will be indicative of the paedophile's sexual preferences. It will contain still photographs or video films, depicting scenes or actions by the protagonists which the paedophile most enjoys or finds most arousing.

Some paedophiles will possess material that would not appear indecent. The images are of children wearing swimwear, school uniform or party clothing. The 'indecency' is the thought or fantasy that the paedophile has when looking at these images. The apparently decent images may of course be legal images of past or current victims. Such images may also be collected from various sources – newspapers, magazine articles, children's clothing catalogues or other people's non-abusive-image photographs. Videos or DVDs may depict scenes from children's television programmes such as *Grange Hill, Play School* or 'Programmes for Schools'. Movies are favourites too, such as *Lord of the Flies*, and films produced for the naturist movement.

In the past, material containing indecent images of children has usually been in the form of either still photographs or videos. More recently, such material is commonly found on computer hard disks, Zip disks, CD-ROMs and DVDs. Computers have allowed the paedophile to develop what was a 'way-out clause'. A photograph showing a naked young adult could be computer enhanced and the image of a child's face grafted to the adult's body. This would be known as a pseudo child image. Today, criminal courts ignore the fact that the body may be that of an adult and look at the photograph as a whole. If the image given is deemed by the jury to be that of a child and is indecent, the court will consider the photograph to be an indecent image of a child.

He will have a preference towards children of particular gender, age and possessing specific physical features

In a similar fashion to a person who has an orientation towards adults, a paedophile has preferences for gender, age and physical appearance. As an example, an adult male with an orientation towards adult females may prefer a female who is of Asian origin, between 20 and 25 years of age, having natural dark-coloured hair, between 5'5" and 5'7" tall, of proportionate build but with large breasts, large eyes but a small mouth, speaks quietly and softly, has great intellect and is well educated.

A paedophile will possess preferences concerning the gender, ethnic origin, age (pre-pubescent, pubescent or post-pubescent), build and facial characteristics of his ideal child victim.

It is unlikely that a fixated or a regressed paedophile will have any great concerns about the intellect of his victim. The paedophile may, however, seek children who are either of low intellect or who are mentally disabled or mentally ill, as this may help the paedophile gain greater control over his physically ideal child victim.

It is recognised that the more intellectual and well-organised paedophiles will plan their abuse well in advance. If a paedophile has preferences regarding the age of his victims, the following would be a typical scenario.

The paedophile (let's call him John) likes little girls aged between six and eight years. He is currently abusing two girls (let's call them Jill and Jane), who are both six years of age. As far as John is concerned, he has two years of forthcoming satisfactory abuse with Jill and Jane. In preparation for the time when Jill and Jane become eight years old and no longer of sexual interest to John, John begins looking for possible future victims. He will look for families or single parents of girls who are currently four years of age. He will identify a future child victim (let's call her Susan) and be prepared to spend the next two years working his way into the life of her family. Throughout this period, John will be gently grooming Susan. Susan, on reaching six years of age, will become John's latest victim.

When John's current victims, Jill and Jane, reach the age of eight, the abuse and family interaction will be delicately drawn to a close. Jill and Jane will be left feeling either relieved that the abuse has ended or devastated by the loss of what they may see as their greatest friend. This will of course depend upon the children's view of John and their understanding of what John has been inflicting upon them. John will now begin his abuse of Susan and also begin his search for new future victims.

The older the child he targets, the greater likelihood of him continuing to abuse children of the target's preferred gender

It has been established that paedophiles will generally prefer males *or* females as opposed to both. However, in the world of paedophilia, successful abuse of one's chosen or preferred victim depends largely on the availability of such a victim.

A paedophile who desires a sexual relationship with eight-year-old males but who cannot achieve such a relationship, may well turn his attention to any available female.

The decision of this paedophile to change his direction of abuse will be largely dependent on the paedophile's desperation for sexual activity. If a paedophile has preferences but the desire to achieve sexual gratification is strong, any child in effect 'will do'.

It is also recognised, however, that if a paedophile has a preference for older children (say, males aged 14 to 15 years), he is very likely to maintain his interest in males only (homosexual paedophilia).

It is rare for a fixated paedophile to maintain a sexual relationship with another adult or adults, as sexual attraction towards adults has never developed. However, should this occur then (as is the case with regressed paedophiles) the sexual orientation towards adults is not indicative of the sexual orientation towards children. In short, a male paedophile may maintain a sexual relationship with a female adult while engaging in sexual abuse of a male child.

Use of certain nouns can indicate unhealthy liking towards a child

Paedophiles view children in various forms. The most common is that of being pure, clean and untouched. When paedophiles are describing a child they may well use descriptive words such as *angel, cherub, pure* and *innocent.* The usage of such words by paedophiles may arouse the suspicions of a parent or carer when in conversation with a paedophile.

No precipitating stress or the presence of deteriorating elements required to offend

It must be remembered that the fixated paedophile does not have to suffer a stress-related illness, or undergo a stressful experience, to feel the need to offend. Nor does he have to suffer deteriorating factors in his life such as physical or mental illness, aging, or a breakdown in relationships or reduction in sexual activity with his chosen partner.

References

Freund K. 1990. In 'Pedophilia', Answers.com: www.answers.com/topic/pedophilia #wp-note-20

Hall. 1995. In: 'Pedophilia', Answers.com: www.answers.com/topic/pedophilia#wp-note-31

3

Typical and identifiable behaviour (selection of victims and recognisable methods of grooming)

This section outlines the various common behavioural characteristics displayed by predatory paedophiles when engaged in the active process of 'grooming'. It is vital to accept and remember that a successful paedophile, who will continue to abuse within a family group for many years, will commonly groom the target child, siblings and the child's parents or guardians, long before any physical act is carried out. Invariably, parents and guardians are the first to be groomed.

The majority of active predatory paedophiles develop, through experience, a 'plan of action' or 'behavioural pattern', which is recognised in paedophiliac circles as being common practice. This 'plan of action' or 'behavioural pattern' includes the paedophile's 'grooming profile', which in turn incorporates his 'method of control', and is often unique to the individual paedophile as it develops. In most cases once a paedophile has established and experienced success with a grooming and controlling method, he will continue to use that method time and time again. In doing so, he leaves behind him a recognisable and identifiable 'fingerprint' pattern of behaviour.

Paedophiles who display patterns of behaviour which fall within the parameters of a 'typical paedophiliac profile' expose themselves as offenders or offenders in the making. These identifiable behaviours can be recognised by parents, carers and professionals, if the paedophile is carefully supervised and his activities monitored.

If a child becomes the focus of a paedophile's attention and is targeted for future sexual abuse, some or all of the behaviours, characteristics and methods of grooming listed below may be displayed. Any actions causing concern or suspicion, or reflecting any of the following should be recorded and consideration given to reporting the matter to the authorities.

Using experience, intuition or assistance from other paedophiles, he will select vulnerable children

Paedophiles are very adept at identifying and selecting children who are most likely to be susceptible to persuasive, seductive or threatening behaviour. This may in turn lead to the paedophile having sufficient control of a child to allow for successful sexual abuse. The chosen victims are invariably children who are easily led or too trusting and can often be described as being 'vulnerable'. The paedophile will identify and take advantage of the child's needs, personality and character, and the child's particular family or home circumstances.

Such children may be from family units with low income who do not enjoy the comforts of fancy toys or clothes, or children that are perhaps of low intelligence or have learning difficulties. Children, from whatever background, who have never enjoyed the comfort of having close and loving parents are especially at risk from paedophiles.

Even children who have close and loving parents, who do not have learning difficulties and possess a high level of intellect are not completely safe, as these children may be too trusting and easily led having never had to suffer hardships or unpleasant experiences.

Follows clear patterns of behaviour to make contact with children

A pattern by which a paedophile will work is either learnt through trial and error, founded through learning from immoral websites, or through education from other, successful paedophiles. The networking between paedophiles for both education and contact with potential or established victims can often begin in prison. They learn their skills and practice, like any other proficient, successful offender.

The activity required in establishing contact with an unknown child, or child's group, can take many forms. Some paedophiles will simply loiter in the vicinity of youth clubs, swimming pools or arcades, getting to know the local children and their parents, while at the same time identifying and selecting the most suitable child. Others have been known to create elaborate and intricate schemes to attract or entice children towards them. For some, the Internet provides all that they need – a faceless communication medium, in which an offender can easily mask his true self, creating false names, ages, images and interests. Others choose to present spurious advertisements in the media, responding only to replies most likely to reveal a child's location or contact details.

Will achieve qualifications and status to have greater access to children

Paedophiles have been known to devote years of their lives to academic study in order to graduate in the field of education, thus becoming teachers and holding positions of respected authority. In many cases, such paedophiles have focused on teaching sport-related subjects, with the obvious result of having contact with children in changing rooms, swimming pools and gymnasiums, where often 'hands-on' educational contact is normally accepted. Irrespective of the teaching topic, the position of 'teacher' presents the paedophile with credibility, authority; trust and, above all, allows them an almost inexhaustible flow of potential victims.

Some have joined youth groups and trained for years to become instructors, moving from one boy group to another, either to find new potential victims, or when their paedophiliac activities have identified them as a possible risk to children and they have been forced to move on.

It is therefore necessary to accept that an active paedophile will go to any length and use any means possible to forge a relationship with parents and children alike, in an effort to gain control of a potential child victim.

May be a leader, assistant, secretary, chairman or play any other role within a children's organisation

The easiest way for a paedophile to gain access to children, particularly while children are not under the close careful supervision of their parents or guardians, is by being involved with children's clubs. By holding a position of youth worker, be that as a youth-club leader, club chairman, secretary or even as a fundraiser, the paedophile is in a position of perceived authority and trust. Often, youth clubs arrange events where children will be away from the family home overnight and therefore very vulnerable to the paedophiliac club worker.

A youth-group worker who has, within a relatively short period of time, worked in a number of separate youth groups whose themes differ, e.g. marching bands, football, tennis, cadet forces, dancing, canoeing, church youth, cycling, etc., may be more interested in associating with children for personal sexual purposes than for associating with children to assist with their educational or recreational development.

Paedophiles will also seek positions within other children's groups, such as: children's orchestras, out-of-school educational groups, babysitting circles, children's Internet news groups and many others. A frighteningly large number of paedophiles who are successful in their illegal activities seek positions of trust where they will have unsupervised one-to-one contact with a child. These sought-after positions may be of paid employment or voluntary work, and could include acting as a swimming instructor, a tennis coach or as a personal educational tutor.

History of affiliation with numerous boy groups and unexplained circumstances for changes in membership

Youth groups, for obvious reasons, give rise to a countless number of possible victims. Once established as a leader or volunteer worker, the active paedophile can exert a variable degree of control over the movements, isolation and behaviour of a child. It is for these reasons that youth clubs of all descriptions are among the highest number of paedophiliac-targeted groups of young people. Most non-offending youth workers possess a particular subject interest in which they are experienced. They derive gratification in making their knowledge or skills accessible to others and assist in the development of others, in their chosen interest. It is therefore fairly safe to assume that most non-offending workers remain affiliated to one boy club for a prolonged period without suspicion or raising concern.

For the paedophile, the interest is not the activity provided by the club, but the youthful protagonists involved. Some paedophiles study a particular subject or interest in great depth and have a high level of knowledge about it. One would therefore expect them to remain in that field. However, access to children is the key to a paedophile's success and therefore the transfer from one interest to another is not uncommon. Below are a number of reasons why a paedophile may have a history of affiliation to numerous boy clubs.

- After joining a club as a worker and seeking to establish potential victims, he observes that his sexual preferences cannot be met as the club members are of undesirable ages, race, physical descriptions or intellect.

- Preliminarily joins a youth club but is dissuaded from pursuing commitment due to the comprehensive, in-depth and excellent child protection policy established within the club.
- After receiving a number of complaints concerning inappropriate behaviour, he decides to leave the club before the authorities become involved or parents and local people are made aware of his identity, thus keeping a low profile within the community.

May abuse his authority, or presumed authority, to seduce or control a child

A child may feel safe in the company of an adult if the adult presents himself as a figure of authority. Authority can so easily give a false impression of trust-worthiness. Such authority may come from a paedophile's high position or office within the community. The paedophile may be a teacher, council official, magistrate, member of the clergy, police officer, doctor, youth worker, celebrity or local personality – in fact, any position that a child understandably would consider has 'power' or 'control' over others.

Another kind of authority often sought by the paedophile is that which is unwittingly given to the paedophile by the child's own parent/s or guardian. This 'assumed' authority can be brought about by the parent's welcoming, acceptance and edification of the paedophile and allowing him to supervise the child-victim.

Develops relationships and acceptance with known 'child protection arena' officials

Most sexual abusers of children are constantly on the lookout for personal edification and acceptance within any social or private group. Abusers with experience of grooming adults, and possessing extreme confidence in doing so, will not shy away from associating with unsuspecting professionals who work within the child protection arena. Such abusers recognise that professionals within the child protection arena give knowing friends and family members a sense of security and surety when the professional is in contact with their children. It therefore follows that if a child protection professional is unwittingly friendly with an abuser, the abuser may well be considered not to be a threat as he has been socially accepted by the professional. It is understandable that a parent would place trust in a social worker, police officer or probation officer working within child protection, or a professional with child protection responsibility, and trust the official's judgement in selecting friends or family members with whom he or she associates.

In addition, an extremely confident and perhaps arrogant abuser may attempt and accomplish successful sexual abuse of a child protection official's offspring. This may be as an act of vengeance towards officialdom, a psychologically stimulating challenge or an added sexual thrill.

Has had numerous jobs involving association with children

As offending paedophiles are exposed in any given environment, they move on to new territories and none more so than in employment. Some employing and voluntary organisations have safety precautions such as lists of people whom it would be inappropriate to employ. Local authorities are one such body that maintain lists of people who should not be employed in any situation likely to bring them into contact with children.

Unfortunately, these lists are not always shared between organisations and offenders can slip through the net. As an example, an exposed paedophiliac school bus driver may well gain employment with another bus company providing school transport in a different county. Circulation of the names of inappropriate people has greatly improved in recent times, resulting in offending paedophiles looking for other areas of employment where the 'list' will not impact upon them. This causes a change of theme in their working career. As an example, it is not uncommon for a fully qualified sports teacher to change career direction and become a children's entertainer. This may be followed some years later with another change of career, to that of a nurse, later specialising in paediatrics.

Unexplained circumstances for changes in employer

Work history may be shady or inconsistent. References and employment records may have unexplained gaps. These of course may well be due to periods of imprisonment or other such incarceration, but are more likely to be because employment has been brought to a sudden end by the employer and the paedophile's wishes to keep the reason for the termination to himself.

By his words and actions, portrays himself as a genuine and nice man

We all have a stereotypical 'paedophile' in our mind's eye. I will not attempt to describe all the probable characteristics of such an individual, but I will state that the real danger comes not from the man we immediately recognise as the likely 'perv', but from the 'nice man next door'. To a paedophile, the focus, the priority, the goal, the prize could be your child. A paedophile sees your child as you may see your 'ideal sexual partner'. Think how nice you could be to the person you most want to have a sexual encounter with. Think how nice you could be to that person's friends or family members in order to make the 'ideal person's' acquaintance. Think about the 'extra mile' that you have travelled to be in favour with your current partner. An active paedophile, *with his eye on your child*, will become your 'nice, best friend' if he can.

Establishes friendship with parents/guardian

If making contact with a selected child is not possible through a club, school or activity, etc., or if the paedophile believes that the child is well protected by their parent/s or guardian, then the paedophile may initially set out to deliberately gain the trust of the child's parent/s or guardian before any attempt is made to 'groom' the victim.

A paedophile, having identified a possible victim, may well set out to establish a friendship with one or both of the parents or the guardian prior to any form of contact with the potential victim, e.g. meet and develop friendship at clubs, pubs, night school, place of work, etc., and portray a 'like' interest such as cars, sports, computers, gardening or even ornithology. A targeting paedophile will approach unsuspecting parents or carers and display a false interest in a subject in the hope that the subterfuge can be used as a tool to assist in the infiltration of a chosen family. If necessary a paedophile will learn and study a particular subject, so that they appear learned and convincing when speaking with the parents of a potential victim.

In addition, he may well sympathise with your problems and offer help and support, take your side in an argument or discussion, lend you money, lend you his car, fix a fuse or put up shelves. In short, in your mind he will become a jolly nice and helpful man. Someone you can rely on and call upon for help. Someone you can trust.

May develop a relationship and marry a single mother

An obvious and common goal for a targeting paedophile is to develop a relationship with a single mum – in some cases, entering into marriage. In such situations, the paedophile is presented with unobstructed access to the 'wife's' children and, in doing so, adopts an almost instant authority over them. While offending, the paedophile will maintain a healthy sex life with the victim's mother so as to 'present' himself as a normal man. He will act like a good husband and draw little attention to any perverse sexual behaviour.

Others have married women who do not have children, and together have raised a family of their own, all in an effort for the paedophile to conceal his true nature. It is not uncommon for the paedophile in this circumstance to pose little or no threat to his children, but be an extreme risk to others.

The experienced paedophile will gain favour by gestures such as paying gas, electricity or other amenity bills, offering to reduce the burdens placed upon the parent by helping out with the washing, shopping and ironing. He may even offer to baby-sit or take the children swimming! He will set out to become indispensable. However, single parents are not the sole targets for a paedophile seeking entry into a family unit; mum, dad, grandparents and the children can be taken in by the experienced, well-organised, plausible paedophile.

It is fairly easy for a paedophile to identify the interests of other men and women. Having identified the common interest, the paedophile will be enthusiastic about the topic and may well invite unsuspecting parents to their home to engage in discussion about the subject, or share the showing of photographs about it. This will all take place solely to increase the level of friendship and reduce any barrier that may exist between them.

Becomes indispensable

Invariably, indispensability is a precise and gradual concept used by many paedophiles that choose to target single parents. In many cases, single parents, particularly those with more than one child, are very busy, tired, stressed, financially insecure and ill-supported individuals who are very often grateful for a pleasant, reliable helping hand. Single parents, therefore, are common targets, often being very vulnerable and easily susceptible to the false kindness and insincerity of the targeting paedophile.

The early stages of developing indispensability are simple. It begins with basic support such as helping with cleaning and washing, little odd jobs or DIY about the home, cooking, shopping and other similar mundane household chores that are indicative of common domesticity. As time passes the 'apparently earnest' help becomes more in-depth and has a greater impact upon the single parent's life, making day-to-day living more enjoyable and less arduous. There are outings for the parent and children – clothes, a DVD player, furniture, kitchen appliances, a car, toys, and other means of improving their lifestyle, are 'freely' provided by the paedophile – but, most important of all, bills are paid. Debt is reduced and cleared. The bank balance for once is in the black. The future looks good. The parent feels supported; she and her children are cared for and are financially stable. The paedophile, 'her man', is proving to be good and life without him would be hard to bear as the thought of returning to those dark and hard days is horrifying.

The paedophile is now well on his way to securing a safe environment in which to offend. A number of reasons exist as to why the paedophile is now in a good position to commence the grooming of the children. The following are a number of these reasons.

- The children see their mother trusting and welcoming this man into their (the family's) lives, so therefore they follow their mother's lead and trust him also.
- The children see their mother happy and contented (possibly for the first time in many years) and would not wish to spoil her happiness by reporting any upsetting or inappropriate behaviour, or even abuse.
- If the abuse is minor, the value of the gifts, outings, improved lifestyle, etc., for the children may seem to them a reasonable and acceptable trade-off.
- If the children do complain, the parent may decide that she will ignore the complaints as life is too good with this man and she cannot afford to lose his support.
- A small number of known cases have shown that some single mothers are in such need of financial support, they will engage in a relationship with a man to whom they are not physically nor emotionally attracted, solely to secure financial stability. Finding sexual contact with this chosen man undesirable, they become only too willing to accept the paedophile's sexual abuse of their children – ignoring the pain and suffering their children endure in order to maintain a good personal financial position and improvements in lifestyle.

Note
It is imperative to remember that, in the example above, a single father is wholly capable of being equally susceptible, influenced and selfish.

Portrays fictitious parenthood to gain social acceptance and trust

Some offenders gain trust and acceptance with parents and carers of children by pretending to be parents themselves. They fabricate stories of children they claim to be theirs and carry photographs of children, which are either stolen or are of, for example, nieces or nephews. They will have a detailed and well-versed explanation as to why the children are not with them at present – usually claiming that they are a divorced parent and the mother has taken the children to a far-off location.

Other paedophiles present their home as that of a family dwelling – claiming to be catering for children from their broken marriage, they will have bedrooms in the home that are decorated and furnished for children, and filled with used toys so as to add to the subterfuge.

Makes plans for future availability of victims and takes time to form relationships with children

In an 'Ideal Paedophiliac World', the paedophile will have unlimited access to his preferred victim (although the paedophile will often not consider the child to be a victim). If, as an example, the paedophile prefers boys between the ages of nine and 11, and is currently abusing male (A), he may well identify a future victim (B) while (B) is seven years old. The paedophile may well conduct 'grooming' activities over a period of two years until such time as (A) becomes too old, and (B) becomes the right age, to be attractive to the paedophile. At this point, the whole process may begin again with a new future victim – victim (C).

Learns to pay attention to children, thus making them feel special

Paedophiles will spend great amounts of their time listening to children, particularly to those that receive little attention from parents or carers. The paedophile will pay attention to anything that the child says and make the child feel important by giving credibility both to the child and to what the child has to say.

Some paedophiles will identify the likes and dislikes of a selected child and will go to great lengths to provide the child with whatever he or she likes, causing the child to believe that he or she is an important person in the paedophile's life. The paedophile will exploit the fact that the parents of his 'targeted' child either can't afford or will not provide the various possessions or activities the child so desperately seeks.

Paedophiles will offer such things as car rides to and from social events, school, or clubs, etc.; they will supply toys, computer games, clothes and money. In addition, and much more concerning, is the supply of adult-themed gifts such as make-up, lingerie, cigarettes, illegal drugs, alcohol and X-rated videos. These are readily supplied to children as they help make the child feel grown-up and accepted as a mature person, doing mature things. They, of course, have a secondary, more sinister role; make-up and provocative clothing may arouse the abuser further, illegal drugs and alcohol will lower the child's resistance or inhibitions to physical or sexual acts, and pornographic material may arouse the child or, at the very least, be another facet to lowering the child's sexual inhibitions.

Seeks to portray his actions as normal

A paedophile seeking to gain control of his chosen victim may well set out to convince the innocent and naive child that what they are doing together is completely normal; that sexual activity between adults and children is 'the done thing' and that non-participation in such activities is abnormal and therefore likely to cause the child to be an outcast and ostracised. The paedophile will try to make the child believe that he is carrying out similar activities with other children, but that the behaviour is something that is never discussed with others.

May have pictures, decor, games or adult material in his home that is appealing to children and may use adult pornography to lower the inhibitions of children

Some paedophiles will offer their own homes as places for children to meet and use as they wish. Initially, the paedophile may allow children to go to his house in his absence. This may increase the child's confidence and the belief that the paedophile is harmless and well-meaning. The child will become comfortable within the house and, if problems of any sort arise between the child and parent, the house may become a safe haven, a retreat or a place of sanctuary. The house also becomes a place of fun, of entertainment and pleasure, probably equipped with computer or other electronic games and music systems.

In such circumstances, the paedophile will often encourage visiting children to take drugs and alcohol. This serves to lower a child's inhibitions or ability to resist either physical or psychological control.

In addition, adult pornographic material may be shown and used by the paedophile in a variety of ways:

- The paedophile may use it to rouse the interest of the children in sexual matters. He may use the pornography for his own purposes (masturbation in front of the children).
- He may use it to reduce the inhibitions that a child may have about sex.
- It may also be used during a later stage of the 'grooming process' as a sexual stimulus for the uncertain and inhibited child.

Eventually, the house, and the lifestyle on offer there, forms part of the child's everyday existence and may even become an addiction. The paedophile, still viewed as well-meaning and harmless, now has an almost captive audience. The offering of money, cigarettes, drugs and adult material increases. The child sees the paedophile as a friend, a supplier of 'bad but good' things that to the child, at this point, are acceptable. The paedophile is a source of all that the child should not have, and all within a safe, familiar, and pseudo-adult environment.

The security and privacy afforded by the house, along with disinhibiting alcohol or drugs, may encourage the visiting children to experiment in sexual activity. Initially this may be between themselves. The paedophile may begin his involvement by being an observer so that the children become used to his presence during sexual activity.

Later, through seduction, bribery, coaxing, the threat of withdrawing the alcohol or drugs, or through the threat of violence, the offending paedophile will begin to involve himself in the children's sexual activity.

Drives a wedge between child and parent and adopts a pseudo-parental role

It is very common for the parents of children between the ages of 11 and 15 to be in a constant battle of wills. The child, influenced by peer pressure and the modern aspects of society, invariably wants many things that the average parent sees as 'unfit' or 'inappropriate'. This presents the paedophile with a great opportunity to win favour with a child and undermine parental authority. The paedophile will aim to be the provider of everything which the parents of a child will not allow.

If a parent refuses to provide a child with more money to spend on clothes or travel to the usual meeting places, etc., the paedophile will provide the money. If the parent does not give the ideal birthday or Christmas gift, the paedophile will provide it. The paedophile, by becoming a 'model' provider, may become thought of as a second father figure, and a wedge begins to be driven between the child and its parents.

Another aspect of the pseudo-parent role is that of giving love and attention. Very often in today's hectic world, children do not receive the amount of attention that they crave from their parents. Parents also, trying to do things right, will quite correctly scold or punish their children when necessary, which may cause a degree of short-term animosity within the family group. The well-practised paedophile will identify such situations and will again attempt to become a second father figure, telling the child that he loves him or her. He will offer comfort and support, cuddling the child and seeming to be genuinely concerned about the child's feelings. He will tell the child that his or her real parents do not love them and do not really want them. He will cause the child to feel insecure within the family unit, thereby creating a situation where he, the paedophile, becomes the 'rock' to which the child may cling.

Enjoys the company of children and photographing them

The vast majority of paedophiles, irrespective of their intentions, genuinely enjoy the company of children. They may surround themselves with numerous children, upon whom they will never physically offend. This will be for any one of the following reasons:

- sexually aroused by the mere sight or sounds of children
- will memorise the facial features of children and later masturbate fantasising with the images within his mind
- will have a preferred fantasy developed and needs a fresh supply of children to place within his fantasy
- by having a photograph of a child, he does not have to rely on his ability to remember the image of the child
- can utilise the image in the photograph over and over again
- children generally like being photographed and if a specific child is happy being photographed by an individual (unknown by the child to be a paedophile), there is likelihood that the paedophile will be able, during a later stage of successful grooming, to photograph the child indecently.

Will go to great lengths to isolate children from parents/adults, appearing to 'put himself out' and therefore enhancing his 'nice guy' image

Another example is when a paedophile has worked his way into a single-parent family where the mother is busy, stressed or tired. In such circumstances, he will offer to take the child out for a day, thus giving her a welcome break. Away from the protection afforded by the mother, the paedophile has complete control over the child.

This action has two significant advantages for the paedophile:

1   He has complete control over the child and is therefore able to impose any of the typical grooming methods (fear, bribery, blackmail, etc.).
2   It gives the mother the belief that he is a nice man, always willing to help and support her.

He may not engage in full penetrative sexual intercourse, but prefer a limited physical/sexual involvement

Sexual gratification is largely achieved through psychological excitement, therefore the paedophile may only wish to see the child either dressed or naked and masturbate at a later date with the image of the child in his mind. He may wish to engage in mutual masturbation with the child, or be satisfied solely by the child performing oral sex on him. Many sex offences are power related, and for some paedophiles the grooming period or the control aspect may be all they desire.

Throughout the actively abusing period of a fixated or regressed paedophile's life, he may be responsible for a large number of child molestations

As paedophilia is an orientation, therefore not curable, only controlled, a paedophile will 'want' to abuse whenever possible, probably for the duration of his life.

A paedophile who has studied or learnt the skills necessary to sexually abuse without detection (unbelievably, these skills are written down and available through Internet sites) may well abuse a child and be satisfied that his actions have not and will not be revealed. The paedophile will have gained confidence and will abuse again. His abusing will continue and the number of victims will increase.

Paedophiles that are identified as having a 30-year history of sexually abusing children leave a trail of devastation behind them. Today, many victims of historic abuse are still quietly suffering. A fixated or a regressed paedophile will continue to abuse even after detection and imprisonment.

By associating or networking with other paedophiles, he may create a 'group' of victims

The sharing of information, for some paedophiles, is of great importance, and often their lifeline. While some paedophiles will focus on one victim at any one time and spend months, even years, developing a situation whereby they can successfully abuse the chosen victim, others will prefer to have a number of victims that are readily and routinely available. The development of such a group of victims may be achievable for the sole paedophile, but most likely will be achieved through association or networking; this often occurs following imprisonment.

The seductive paedophile works alone

Although many paedophiles will develop a network of associates for the circulation of information, photographs or indeed children, many will also work alone when initially targeting a child or when establishing a friendship with the targeted child's family.

Possesses a history of indecent exposure convictions

Many paedophiles start their sexual offending career by indecently exposing themselves to children. This is classed as a 'non-contact' sexual offence. Stimulation and/or arousal will commence as a result of seeing a child; further sexual excitement will be generated as a result of exposing their penis to a child. Following on from the exposure is sexual climax, which is likely to occur later when the paedophile masturbates, recalling and fantasising over the incident.

Do not be fooled by those paedophiles that claim they 'only look at pictures' (another non-contact sexual offence)

First, it is important to realise that indecent images of children can exist in various forms. They can be:

- unedited photographs (Polaroid/self-produced images from photographic negative)
- unedited images in specifically produced magazines
- images produced as a collage (an innocent image of a child with an image of adult genitalia pasted on top forming an indecent pseudo-image of a child, or an innocent image of a child with an image of a naked adult pasted next to it; the overall content of the combined image can be deemed to be indecent)
- unedited images stored/downloaded on a computer (the image, stored as a digital code, is considered to be the same as a photographic image). Possession of such an image stored as a digital code is considered to be 'possession of indecent material'. Transforming that digital code to an image either on the computer screen or into a printed photograph is considered to be 'making indecent material'
- edited images – computer-edited/grafted images (an image made up of a naked adult's body and a child's face is considered to be an indecent pseudo-image of a child)
- edited or unedited video (VHS) film/computer video clips.

Many paedophiles convicted of possessing indecent images of children will tell you that they are not paedophiles, as they have not been charged with, or convicted of, indecently assaulting or raping a child and have therefore never touched or hurt a child. They will tell you that they do not pose any physical threat to children. They may; they may not. The true level of risk they pose to children can only be fully assessed by a suitably qualified professional: some individuals guilty of possessing such material pose significant risk; others do not. It is worthy to note that if no evidence exists to prove an act of physical sexual abuse on a child by an individual, then equally no evidence will exist to prove that the individual has *not* physically sexually abused a child.

'You only collect things in which you have an interest.' A man who collects indecent images of children does so because he has a sexually explicit interest in children. It is not uncommon for the police to seize indecent material from an offender and find hundreds or even thousands of indecent images of children. When computers are seized from suspects and the data storage interrogated, the audit trail can show that thousands of such images have been downloaded and either stored on the hard disk, downloaded to other storage (floppy disk, memory stick or CD-ROM) or deleted once viewed.

The interesting point with stored images is that they indicate the true preference of a paedophile. On average, 60–70% of a paedophile's collection will be that of his preferred gender, race and age range of victims. The collection will also indicate the type of preferred activity. If, for example, the majority of images stored by a paedophile show Asian females aged between 9 years and 11 years of age, all being forced to interact sexually with adult males, it is highly likely that the paedophile's sexual preference is that of 9- to 11-year-old Asian females, and his fantasy or desire is that of engaging in sexual activity with them.

Research has shown, however, that not all paedophiles that derive satisfaction from viewing indecent images of children move on to indecently assaulting or raping children. It is true, though, that 98% of sexual abusers of children have, at some time prior to their physical offending, viewed indecent images of children.

With the current legal and social stance on paedophilia in the United Kingdom, paedophiles who are in the position to do so will view indecent images of children while residing in the UK, and travel abroad to conduct their 'contact sexually abusive offending'.

Will utilise his children as 'tools' to make contact with other children

Paedophiles who have become fathers often use their children in many illegal and immoral ways. First, their children may become victims themselves. This depends of course upon the gender and age of the child and the paedophile's sexual preference. Second, a paedophiliac father, with a sexual preference for boys aged between five and seven years, may encourage his nine-year-old son to befriend younger children, who in turn may become future victims. Conversely, a paedophiliac father may encourage his younger children to befriend and associate with older children.

Claims not to like children or requests that children are kept at a distance; later, becomes involved with the very same children

On entering a community or housing complex, a paedophile may well express to other residents, both with or without children, that he does not like children and wish they would all stay away from him and give him peace. This is an acceptable request and plea especially for a man in his later years, and so other residents are quickly duped into believing that the paedophile genuinely wants to distance himself from local children. This will assist the paedophile in establishing acceptability and credibility within the community and give him the appearance of normality.

He may well, at a later stage, play the martyr and have children in his company, along with the parents or carers initially, playing the role of the 'put-upon old man' that is helping out. The paedophile will watch carefully and identify parents and carers who are perhaps 'struggling' with time and money. He may well, when he feels the time is right, offer to assist with childminding or shopping. This will help to develop a greater friendship between the paedophile and the selected parent, and may also create a situation where the parent becomes a little reliant upon the paedophile. The targeted parent will feel confident that the paedophile has little or no interest in children and will be more likely to be prepared for his or her child to be cared for or supervised by the paedophile.

Discloses early in relationship his cautions or convictions for child sex abuse, claiming to be innocent

A ploy used by many convicted paedophiles is to disclose convictions of child sexual assault almost immediately upon entering a new relationship, claiming to have been wrongfully accused, harassed and 'fitted-up' by the police, prejudiced by the legal services and the courts, etc. – the aim being to convince the new friend that he must be innocent: '. . . *why else would a man tell me this at this stage if it weren't true . . . ?*' Once the new friend is convinced and successfully groomed, she is unlikely to believe any account or warning given by others, even the police or social services, as to the paedophile's likelihood of offending against her children.

Specific targeting of disabled children

Children with a physical or a mental disability or both

It is imperative to remember that a disability experienced by one child can so clearly be very different from a disability experienced by another. Therefore, the level of vulnerability will vary accordingly. A child with acute physical disability is at risk in a very different way from a child with learning or communication difficulties.

A child with a mental or physical disability or both is extremely vulnerable to the abusive actions of a paedophile and more easily abused due to any one of the following.

- A child suffering a severe mental disability may have communication difficulties and not be in a position to inform genuine carers of historic or current abuse.
- A physically or mentally disabled child may not possess sufficient physical ability or mental capacity to resist or shun abuse.
- They may be totally isolated from other children or may have fewer friends or associates with whom to confide and discuss normal activities. Therefore, they fail to identify that the actions of an abuser are wrong, immoral and illegal.
- They may receive close and/or intimate personal physical care, which may be an opportunity for the paedophiliac carer to take advantage of. In addition, the child may well have numerous carers, which may cause confusion, uncertainty and identification difficulties if abuse is reported.
- They may be vulnerable to humiliation and intimidation by non-disabled children and therefore more likely to cling to and accept the friendship of a person showing support and understanding.

- They may be incapable of understanding or recognising the actions of the abuser as being abusive.
- A child suffering with a minor mental disability may be unable to cope with the pressure and trauma experienced while either disclosing the abuse to a third party, or appearing in a court of law even when protected by video link.

Will use his own, a relative's or friend's disabled child to gain favour and sympathy from other parents and make further contact with children

Gaining sympathy, giving the appearance of being a kind and caring person, acting as the martyr and playing the part of a down-trodden, weak individual are some of the methods used by paedophiles to obtain from parents aspects such as acceptance, friendship, credibility, tolerance and support. There is no better way of achieving these benefits than spuriously presenting oneself as the hard-working, under-pressure, apparently devastated carer of a physically or mentally disabled child.

Various scenarios outlining typical paedophiliac usage of disabled children

Child with under-developed mental age

A paedophiliac father with a 14-year-old son, with a mental age of nine, can be used to make friends with nine-year-old children and draw them to the family home.

Associates with parents of other disabled children

An active paedophile may well join clubs or support groups, which offer child-care, or respite to parents, thereby gaining access to disabled children.

The benefits open to a paedophile caring for a disabled child are numerous. In addition to the above, the benefits include:

- gains access to specialist schools and homes for disabled children
- gains control of disabled child-victim with greater ease and may involve child-victim in sexual abuse with other disabled victims so that the child-victim sees other children engaging (unwillingly) in sexual activity and accepts this behaviour as normal
- gains sympathy from parents and carers of both disabled and able-bodied children
- gains credibility and greater social standing by portraying the role of a caring, honest man, who may have given up work or other normal activity to care for his child
- gains acceptance in the 'disabled child-caring' social arena
- gains access to other disabled children, where the paedophile may well offer or be asked to care for disabled children of others
- gains the position of an 'innocent party' should a complaint of sexual abuse be made, by dispelling responsibility and placing blame on a disabled child – this is particularly used when a child with a mental disability is involved.

Various scenarios outlining typical paedophiliac subterfuge – based on known cases and cases reported by the media

Studies photography, portrays himself as a photographer, advertises photographic services

One offender studied photography at night school and became an accomplished photographer advertising a specialist knowledge and ability to photograph children for modelling and catalogue work. In an effort to increase the flow of children attending his studio, he would falsify photographic contracts and modelling work, advertising under various company names. Apart from the obvious opportunities to photograph children in underwear, swimwear and light summer clothing, he also indulged in 'child glamour' photography, convincing parents that glamour-type photographs of their child would catch the attention of modelling agencies and agents. The glamour photographs made children appear as young adults and assisted the offender in the process of cognitive distortion.

In addition, he produced thousands of pseudo-abusive images of children by digitally grafting the images of a child's face onto an image of a young adult's naked body.

Children's entertainer

A fairly obvious and well-used method of gaining access to children is by way of purporting to be a children's entertainer. Offenders can take the guise of a mobile disco operator, a magician, arts and craft instructor, rare musical instrument teacher or a puppeteer.

Among the most common of these guises are magicians and disco operators, often providing amusement for children at schools, play groups, family fun days and at nurseries. It is not uncommon for offenders opting for these methods to establish themselves within school and community childcare circles, as well as being recommended to many families or child groups.

The method of offending can vary, but often such offenders utilise the aspect of being the centre of attention as an opportunity to be physically close to children or to obtain indecent photographs or indecent video footage of children.

Offenders have used numerous ways of surreptitiously obtaining indecent images of children and one such method has been to secrete covert still image and video cameras inside magician lecterns or inside mobile disco speakers at floor level. The offenders have then been found to arrange children in such a way as to be seated 'cross-legged', directly in front of the lectern or speakers, usually with the girls sitting in front of the boys. The offender would then activate the cameras by remote switch and take indecent photographs of the children.

One offender, utilising the mobile disco option, had mounted a remote control strobe and laser light unit on a pole; the unit could be moved up or down the pole to any height. The light unit had been adapted to conceal a camera, which was also activated by remote control.

Some children's entertainers will overtly video-record children at the event, claiming they are producing a 'promotional video'.

Will present himself as a disabled person

Many people naively believe that a man in a wheelchair poses little risk of harm to a child – after all, he cannot chase a child, he cannot easily force himself upon a child, and most likely does not appear imposing or intimidating. In addition, few people will question the validity of someone sitting in a wheelchair.

Most of us will assume that the wheelchair user is physically disabled unless they are bandaged or in plaster. This is a totally reasonable and usually correct assumption. It is not always a safe assumption to make. One such person, presenting himself in public and at court in a wheelchair, was found to be physically able, and could easily walk. He has no physical disability, yet for years convinced doctors, social workers, neighbours, teachers and children that he could not stand. His plausibility and subterfuge was so good, he even duped a credible 'disabled vehicle' support charity into providing him with a car.

Another offender with a series of convictions for sex attacks on children presented himself as a disabled man, needing the support of a wheelchair. He has, while in his chair, used the threat of violence, physically held a child against his will, committed a number of serious indecent assaults and assaulted police officers. In addition, he has used his 'disabled' position to gain access to areas of schools, play areas and family fun events to which the majority of the public would not be given access. He regularly manipulates adults into feeling sorry for him and acting in a supportive and helping fashion. He has even coerced parents into sending their children to him, to help with his garden, house tidying and to read to him. Many of these children have suffered sexual assaults.

Simple advertising

One offender placed an advert in a London paper inviting contact with a view to marriage from single mothers of blue-eyed, fair-haired boys. He received eight replies and married a young single mother. Throughout the ensuing 30 years of marriage, he and his 'advertised wife' fostered over 200 children, most of whom he abused until he was caught and prosecuted at the age of 63 (Wyre 1998).

Children's and youth-club worker

Numerous male offenders affiliate themselves to children's and youth clubs. The reason is fairly obvious – to gain contact with a consistent flow of a large number of children. An added advantage for the paedophile is that by careful selection of an appropriate club, the paedophile can choose the age range of child with whom he will come into contact. The majority of clubs, be they general sports clubs, church clubs (Boys' and Girls' Brigade, etc.), scouts, armed forces cadet clubs, marching bands, specialist activity clubs (astronomy, writing, conservation, computer study, etc.), do not specialise in providing services for severely disabled children. Clubs offering such a resource will be of particular interest to paedophiles that are focused on offending against disabled children; however, being specialist clubs, it is likely that they will only draw interest from paedophiles that have attained knowledge and experience in a club's particular specialist theme.

Understandably, clubs attracting the general attention of paedophiles are clubs which, by their very nature, encourage child members to leave the safety of the family home for one or more nights, sleeping either alone or with other children under the supervision of the club's leaders and workers.

Sporting clubs are particularly attractive to paedophiles. This is primarily due to the acceptance that many tutoring aspects call for direct physical contact between coach and player, and that a sporting coach would not be out of place frequenting changing areas or showers. In addition, many sporting clubs engage in competitions which very often call for players and coaches to travel to venues in other towns, sometimes necessitating the need for overnight accommodation.

(It should be noted that many children's sporting clubs have adopted rules which do not allow sports trainers or coaches to be in company with players during changing and showering periods; however, not all clubs have adopted this rule and not all clubs are routinely monitored.)

Children's and youth club worker – example: An offender, whom I shall fictitiously call John, grew up learning the discipline of boxing. This was not unusual at the time of John's youth, but what was unusual was that by the age of 11, John realised that he was sexually attracted to his peer group – other 11-year-old boys. He found that he was not sexually attracted to the adult males who often appeared, as did the boys, naked in the showers and changing rooms, just boys. He pursued his boxing career, not because of the enjoyment of the sport, but as an access to boys of his and similar ages. He continued his affiliation with his club into adulthood and until a small number of boys complained about incidents of inappropriate behaviour. Neither he nor the incidents were reported to the authorities, and after discussions with the club organisers he simply left his club and joined another boxing club in the same city. Rumours abounded, but still the authorities were not informed. Motivated and encouraged by the fact that neither officials within the clubs nor members were reporting his activities, he spread his area of activity and joined other boys' and sporting clubs. For three decades, John has immersed himself in boy work, associating with children from all backgrounds and overseeing them on overnight sporting events, giving one-on-one tuition in boxing and other disciplines.

His 'planning' part of the offending-cycle process would begin by developing regular, friendly, supportive and unsuspicious contact with a group of about eight to ten boys. He would always pay particular attention to the same group so as to isolate them from all others. Within this group, John would select one individual that he thought most likely to best respond to the grooming process. He would provide all the boys in the group with equal gifts and money and take them all, in small groups, out for meals and shopping trips. Each boy felt that he was being treated like all the others. John would then focus his attention on his chosen boy and begin a protracted, threatening, grooming process. The boy was manipulated into thinking that all the boys in the group were being treated in the same way and so the chosen boy would say nothing. He was forced to perform various sex acts and was 'rewarded' with unwelcome payment, increasing the victim's own feelings of guilt and adding to the threat of exposure as a 'willing participant' of male prostitution.

The process and method of offending was repeated by John, tens if not hundreds of times. It provided a fairly safe environment to offend, as John had the opportunity to select the most suitable victim, the victim was unlikely to speak out due to the controlling fear imposed by John, and if the victim had spoken out, John could deny the allegations and produce eight or ten other boys who would all say that they had been given gifts, etc., but never inappropriately approached, threatened, coerced, manipulated or sexually abused.

Childcare worker

Qualifying and securing employment in an environment where dealing directly, often without supervision, with children with problems (drug or alcohol abusers, psychologically impaired or disturbed, behavioural problems or learning difficulties, etc.) is a very common and successful method of accessing, developing control of, and offending against children. Securing secrecy is made easier if the child suffers from a psychiatric or psychological disability or illness, and denial of offending is easier if the complaining child has a history of substance abuse or behavioural difficulties. Children who are in local authority secure or residential care for criminal offences are also vulnerable as they may be regarded as having little or no credibility, and therefore may not be believed when making allegations of sexual or physical assault.

Some offenders have been gainfully employed in a large number of children's homes, moving from one home to another if complaints are made by children in their care. Sometimes they change their name and history to secure a new position, sometimes slipping through the 'net' of child welfare officialdom.

For some, marriage and short-term foster caring is the answer to their dreams – an almost inexhaustible supply of children who are, by the very nature of being fostered, likely to be upset, vulnerable, timid and effortlessly controlled through fear, highly dependent on others, easily influenced and coerced, possibly corruptible and readily persuaded to perform sex acts for money or other rewards.

Working with vulnerable children presents an adult with a sexual interest in children with the greatest of opportunities to develop and progress on the offending cycle and ultimately commit sexual offences.

Reference

Wyre R. Author's notes from personal attendance at Sex Offender Awareness Training Seminar. West Yorkshire Police Headquarters, Training Department; 1998.

4

What stops a child reporting abuse and pointing out the abuser?

In order for a paedophile to enjoy a lifelong, unhindered and successful career of child sexual abuse, he has to secure an imposed and flawless method of control over all his victims, which will prevent them from 'telling'. The known methods of grooming and control are numerous and varied. In most cases once a paedophile has established and experienced success with a grooming and controlling method, he will continue to use that method time and time again. In doing so, he leaves behind him a recognisable and identifiable 'fingerprint' pattern of behaviour.

Children suffering one or more of the four main types of abuse may have many reasons, simple or complicated, why they will choose, feel compelled or be forced not to inform the authorities, their parents, teachers or friends, of the true nature of the abuse or the abuser. It is important to remember that an abused child may not be in a mental state to assess events and circumstances, or consider appropriate action with any degree of rationality. The ability to ingest and analyse events and think clearly about the issue of disclosure is highly dependent upon the level and success of the grooming imposed and/or the abuse taking place. Throughout the period of grooming and successful abusing, the child may feel completely and totally under the control of the abuser.

Any abused child choosing not to disclose the issue of suffering abuse to others may do so for one or more of the following reasons.

Fear

Fear, in all its forms, is a major weapon used by many paedophiles in their quest to psychologically overpower and control a chosen potential victim. Fear is easy to instil, maintain and deny, as no physical evidence would exist. No physical act need take place as fear can be induced in the child's mind by careful and skilful psychology.

The paedophile will induce fear in the following ways.

- Threatening immediate violence towards the victim should they either fail to comply with his wishes, report the abuse or report the abuser. The threat can be that of a minor assault such as punching or kicking, or can be extreme such as the threatening of life, sometimes showing the victim a knife or firearm to instil greater fear.
- Threatening immediate violence towards the victim's family, should the victim again fail to comply with his wishes, or report the abuse or abuser.

Again the production of weapons can instil greater fear in the victim's mind. Similar threats can also be made towards the victim's friends, associates or even pets.

- Instilling belief in the victim's mind that her parents will be violent towards her if she should 'tell', as parents do not believe their children when they report abuse (this is very often the case when the abuser is a member of the family).
- Instilling belief in the victim's mind that she will be taken away from the family home and placed in care should she report the abuse or abuser. The thought of being isolated from one's own loving parents is terrifying for a child of any age and therefore the abuse remains undetected.
- Instilling belief in the victim's mind that nobody will believe them and that they will be laughed at, ridiculed, ostracised and lose all credibility with family and friends. The feeling of hopelessness and worthlessness may also creep into the victim's mind, especially if the victim thinks there is a possibility that they will not be believed, even by their parents.
- Blackmailing the child by threatening to divulge to others their involvement in drug taking, alcohol use, engaging in sexual activity with other children (even if this is untrue), or any other matter which the child would not want others to know. Rarely will the child realise that should the abuser divulge such information, the abuser himself is likely to be identified as the provider of the materials to which the blackmail is related.

Forcing unwanted payment – made to feel responsible

It is common for paedophiles to enforce a reward upon their victims or potential victims. The practice of rewarding victims and potential victims usually commences during the grooming process, when the paedophile is perhaps acting in an overbearing way or forcing issues of control. The forcing of the acceptance of a reward may, in itself, be considered abusive and acts to reinforce the control and manipulation the paedophile possesses over his victim. In addition, the paedophile may:

- be validating and enforcing his cognitive distortion insomuch as he believes the victim to be a willing, fee-charging participant, and will promote this belief in his victim's mind
- in time cause his victim to feel that they have played an active role in the planning of arrangements to have sex and therefore feel partly or wholly responsible
- reduce his victim's self-worth or self-esteem by creating a situation whereby his victim is made to feel like a prostitute, and will enforce in his victim's mind that 'acting as a prostitute' is exactly how his victim's parents, friends, police or social service workers will view her.

Guilt

The laying of blame is very much a major part of the paedophile's cycle of offending, as it allows the relief of guilt and in some way justifies his illegal and immoral actions. The offending paedophile will often blame his wife for his offending, as he will portray her as failing or not willing to engage in sufficient or satisfactory sex.

He may also blame his behaviour upon having an illness such as depression or alcoholism. He may blame friends for introducing him to abusive or indecent images of children, which has created unwanted and uncontrollable paedophiliac sexual stimulation. However, blame is most commonly laid at the feet of his victim. The paedophile may well tell his victim, with alarming regularity and forcefulness, that she is to blame for the abuse. Continued manipulation and convincing assertiveness may well lead his victim to genuinely believe that she is responsible for the events that have 'gone on' between her and the offender. If the paedophile is successful with this method, he will make his victim carry the burden of guilt for every single matter concerning his abuse of her. He may make her feel guilt about her family and any disruption caused to them, and he may make her feel guilty about the destructive effect that their actions have had upon him and his family, should the abuse become disclosed.

Embarrassment

For most boys, male teenagers and men, it is or would be embarrassing to admit, to a family member, friend, lover or spouse, that he has suffered sexually abusive acts such as buggery or has been forced to perform oral sex upon a man. If given the choice, most male victims who have suffered such atrocities, that have since stopped, choose to refrain from reporting the abuse, electing to 'keep it quiet'.

Family disruption

The victim may well recognise that reporting abuse, especially if the abuser is part of the family group, will bring about tremendous disruption and upheaval. If, for example, the abuser is the 'new man' in the victim's mother's life, the victim may well feel that the abuse is less of a psychological pain than the emotional pain that would be experienced by yet another family break-up.

The victim may also wish for their mother to be happy and may well endure the abuse for the sake of their mother's happiness. On occasions, the relationship between the mother and 'new man' may be such that the victim may feel that reporting abuse will not be readily accepted by the mother and that the victim may well be shunned. It is not uncommon for the mother to 'side' with the abuser, the mother having disbelieved the victim.

The mother may think that the complaint is as a result of jealousy and again it is not uncommon for the mother to choose the 'new man' and remove the victim from the family home.

If the abuser is the father or grandfather, the victim may be too afraid to cause upset within the family, thinking that all the family members will not believe their story and will make life for the victim very unhappy. A similar situation may exist if the abuser is another close family member. As an example, the abuser could be an uncle, perhaps the father's brother. Disclosure of the abuse to another family member, or the authorities, appears not to be an option for the victim as they do not wish to upset the father and cause a breakdown in their father's relationship with his brother.

Personal disruption

Many children who have experienced continual changes in their care, be it temporary foster care, care homes, homelessness or change of carers within the family group, may find themselves in a situation that, for the first time in their life, suits them. It may be a situation in which it appears 'everything is coming together', 'a home they have never had'. The impact for a young child to find him- or herself in such a settled and harmonious position may be so great that the child will not allow anything to disrupt or endanger its continuance, as there is little likelihood of replicating the circumstance.

A skilled and perceptive paedophile may recognise the child's recent happiness and feelings of security and want, and prey upon the child, threatening the existence of the safe haven the child has found.

Love or affection for the abuser

Where the abuser is a family member or a close friend to the victim and the non-abusive aspect of the relationship is valued or is a necessity to the victim, the child in question may well suffer the abuse in silence, continuing to love the abuser. As an example, a daughter may love her father unconditionally, suffering the abuse without complaint – although wishing for the abuse to stop.

Reporting the abuse is not an option for her as she could not bear her father being arrested, sent to prison or not being seen again – the loss of her beloved father is too great. Almost a 'love–hate' relationship exists – she loves her father, but hates him for what he does.

Enjoys the high life

An abuser may well be seductive and provide his victim with a 'dream-like' lifestyle. The victim may be treated to various luxuries such as designer clothing, the latest mobile telephone, being transported around in a 'flash' car, taken to top quality hotels or to enjoy lavish holidays, given cash to spend or even a credit card, or may even be housed in a luxurious apartment. The luxuries, in the mind of the victim, are a reasonable 'trade-off' for the abuse that he or she has to endure. Reporting the abuse would mean an end to the high life. Although this scenario may paint a picture of the victim playing a willing role and even appearing as a prostitute, the victim is still a victim, preyed upon by the seduc-tive paedophile.

Needs the rewards

Some paedophiles, during the 'grooming' period, will introduce the victim to drugs, causing the victim to become an addict. This puts the paedophile into a very strong controlling position. The paedophile can use this situation in one of two ways. First, he can be the 'supplier of the drugs' and receive his remuneration by way of enforced sexual activity, the victim choosing to either go without the drugs or perform sex acts with the abuser or abuser's associates. Second, he can initially supply his victim with drugs without payment until a substantial debt is owed. Suddenly the abuser calls in the debt (usually with menaces) and offers the victim a method by which to clear or reduce the debt. The offer will be to perform minor sex acts with the abuser or abuser's associates. As time passes, the abuse will become more severe, usually resulting in full penetrative sex.

Inability to communicate

Some of the most vulnerable of all children and young people are those who cannot communicate between themselves, with trusted and safe adults, and with the outside world. The reason for their exposure to such high risk is obvious, in that the offender is not required to develop a secure 'non-telling' environment in which to offend. His victim is already silenced. The victim's inability to communicate may lie in a physical or mental impairment, or psychosis; and, as outlined in Chapter 3, individuals requiring close and intimate attention, both in nursing and private care, are often greatly at risk.

The abuser himself may create in the mind of a child-victim such fear that the victim cannot speak – either permanently or, most commonly, when in the presence of the abuser.

Manipulated or unplanned isolation

Restricting the access a victim has to other people is a method of control and security employed by some abusers. Often, such a method is engineered by the helpful 'new man' or relative and can consist of taking the child victim on holiday, or having the child victim reside with the paedophile at his home address.

On occasions, a child victim may become isolated due to unforeseen circumstances such as bereavement within a family group, leaving a father and daughter alone; or a grandson residing with grandparents, open to abuse by the paedophiliac parent or carer.

Police interview/court ordeal

Many child victims, particularly older child victims who simply wish for the sexual (or other) abuse to stop, may refrain from reporting the abuse to the authorities, family or friends, fearing a presumed harrowing police interrogation and the possible ensuing courtroom ordeal. These presumptions are primarily due, unfortunately, to too many television programmes, too many books and too many 'anti-police' barrack-room lawyers having contaminated the minds of many young and older children. This 'unwarranted harmful brainwashing' is in addition to the 'specific and pernicious brainwashing' imposed by the manipulative paedophile that has, most likely, already successfully convinced his victim of issues such as:

'... the police will be hard on you and not believe your story and, even if they do, you will go through hell at court with lots of people staring at you and not believing you ... they will call you a liar.'

Abused children therefore may assume that if they report the abuse, leading to the police and court becoming involved, they will receive harsh and unpleasant treatment, humiliation and, in the end, will not be believed. This could not be further from the truth. All police forces in the United Kingdom, working alongside supporting and social-work agencies, have laboured for many years to develop joint-working practices required to professionally deal with child victims of abuse; 'joint-working practices' provide support, security, comfort and methods of how best to extract evidence from victims. This type of work is now undertaken by specialist and dedicated officers who form Child Protection Units within each police force and local authority. The units are staffed with male and female officers who have received specialised training for working with victims of child abuse. In theory the term 'interrogation', as used above, is correct although it conjures up ideas of a sparsely decorated room with a desk, two chairs and a spot lamp shone into the victim's face. Again, this is wholly unrealistic.

5

Behavioural thought processes – child sex offending (cycle of thought and deed)

It is highly improbable that any one person or group could substantially, with long-term success, combat the sinister process undertaken by an individual paedophile once he has entered a cycle of abusive thought and deed, without possessing an understanding of the process itself.

If child or family healthcare professionals, police officers, social workers, therapists or members of offender support groups are to significantly reduce the risk of a paedophile offending or re-offending, they need to have a clear and an in-depth understanding of the complex and sometimes ritual-like process in which most, if not all, child sex abusers choose to participate. The identical knowledge and understanding applies if the same professional bodies, along with guardians, carers and parents of children, are to protect children from the psychological harm of grooming and the physical suffering of sexual victimisation as is imposed by offending paedophiles.

The 'cycle of thought and deed' process is an addictive continuum; though it may wane from time to time, it will be forever in the mind of the offending paedophile. Breaking or disrupting the cycle is highly unlikely in most cases as only a few are given the opportunity to experience and engage in quality, long-lasting therapeutic treatment.

Even prosecution and imprisonment does little to break or diminish the cycle, as fantasy plays a very large part in the offending process and is obviously an uncontrollable factor, even when in prison. In fact, it could be argued that imprisonment creates a greater threat, as paedophiles rarely receive lifelong custodial sentences. They will, therefore, be circulating in society at some future time in their lives. The fantasies created and repeatedly experienced by imprisoned child sex offenders may well develop into future offences – the concern being that over the period of incarceration the fantasies will increase both in regularity and, more concerning, in sexually deviant severity.

It is often the case that serving child sexual abuse prisoners will establish friendships with either gullible or desperate single female parents while they remain in custody, through writing clubs or a 'prisoner support organisation'. Some of these friendships result in the paedophile being released from prison to a female single parent, waiting outside the prison walls – an almost idealistic situation for the sexually frustrated, skill-honed paedophile with a host of fantasies bursting to be acted out into reality.

For the individual paedophile, the cycle is only broken if the paedophile himself chooses to break it. (*See* Figure 5.1.)

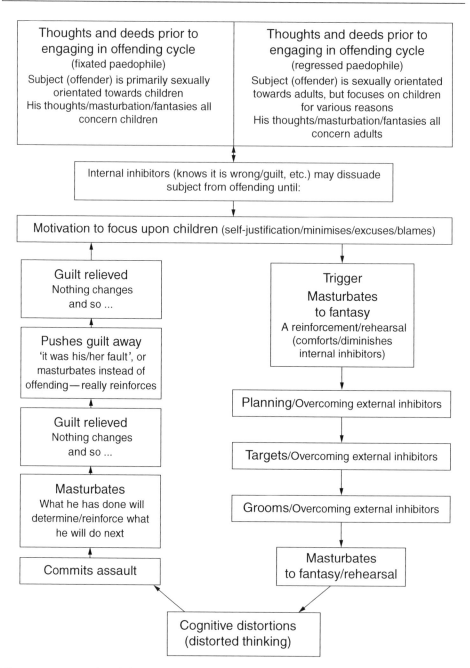

Figure 5.1 Cycle of thought and deed for a man who sexually offends against children.

Thoughts and deeds prior to engaging in offending cycle fixated paedophile

The fixated paedophile, as described earlier in this book, will be sexually orientated towards children. He is unlikely to be sexually or emotionally stimulated by adults and if he has engaged in an emotional and sexual relationship with an adult, he is likely to have done so having suppressed his true feelings and urges for children.

He may continually find his attention being drawn towards children and feel sexually aroused by children. However, in an attempt to refrain from involvement he may turn away, fantasise and masturbate while alone, partake in sexual activity with an adult while fantasising about a child or even secure a relationship with a willing adult partner to role-play as a child.

Thoughts and deeds prior to engaging in offending cycle – regressed paedophile

The regressed paedophile, as described previously, will have lived any amount of his life being sexually and emotionally aroused by adults of either gender, dependent upon the paedophile's initial sexual orientation. Certain life experiences, opportunities, illnesses, etc., may affect the sexual arousal stimulus and the individual becomes sexually and/or emotionally interested in children, both solely or in addition to his initial sexual orientation, thus creating and maintaining what appears as a normal husband/wife (family) existence, but engaging in thoughts of sexual desire of children.

At this stage, he will continue to have his attention drawn to adults whom he recognises as sexually attractive. However, if there is an unlikelihood of him forging a relationship of his choosing with such adults and he acknowledges this fact, he may well fantasise and masturbate – but at this time solely concerning adults.

Internal inhibitors

Internal inhibitors, the paedophile's conscience, will at this stage be reasonably strong. In most cases at this point, both the fixated and regressed paedophile accepts that engineering and carrying out a sexual relationship with a juvenile is wrong. At this time he may experience feelings of self-repulsion at the thought of conducting a sexual relationship with a child and he may even feel guilt concerning the probable physical and emotional harm and suffering he may cause to the child.

Examples of *internal inhibitors*:

- fear – of one's own inability to control distorted thinking and/or perverse sexual desires
- honest denial – not admitting to oneself one's true sexual orientation
- self-repulsion of one's own sexual persuasion and/or desire
- conscience – knowing it to be wrong and wrestling with one's own beliefs of right and wrong.

Motivation to focus upon children (self-justification/ minimises/excuses/blames)

Finkelhor (1986) suggests a number of elements contained in an individual's life that may, when combined, motivate that person to actively engage in behaviour that will lead to the sexual abuse of a child. These elements can be sexual preference (heterosexually, homosexually or bisexually paedophiliac or hebephiliac), emotional and/or behavioural similarity to children (mentally relates and associates with children to an accomplished level), emotional loneliness or being socially ostracised.

Some paedophiles derive motivation from their own, or perceived own, historic child abuse experiences. Many offenders will excuse their paedophiliac behaviour by claiming that 'what was done to me justifies what I do to others'. Though it must be understood and remembered that while an average of 65% of sex offenders (Sullivan 2000/2001) report to have been victims of sexual abuse as children, this does not explain or give rise to justification for becoming an abuser. A large proportion of child sexual abuse victims mature to be satisfactory and sometimes extraordinary spouses and parents.

Many paedophiles are motivated by the belief that children can give meaningful and informed consent for others to violate their bodies. Others firmly believe that God made children for adults to abuse. Some paedophiles convince themselves that they are 'doing the child a favour' by educating the child in sexual matters.

Many times, offending paedophiles will psychologically minimise their illegal sexual fantasy and/or activity. '... I'll only touch her the once ... it happened a long time ago ... it didn't or won't cause any harm ... I didn't hurt him ... she didn't complain so it couldn't have been that bad ...' This only serves to lessen the guilt and the level of responsibility perceived by the offender. When grooming, minimising any previously convicted offences or known behaviour may assist in convincing others that the paedophile was wrongfully or overly held responsible for the illegal sexual acts.

A few will deny that the offending ever took place and may develop an intricate and plausible facade as a cover story. In time the paedophile may well genuinely believe his facade and fail to ever again recognise the truth. Mental disability or mental illness can also be incorporated within the facade. On occasions, paedophiles have been recorded claiming that 'they were led astray by the child' – the child therefore being accused of initiating the sexual activity, hardly likely in cases where the child victim is only four years of age.

Trigger – masturbates to the fantasy. A reinforcing rehearsal (comforts and diminishes internal inhibitors, combats external inhibitors)

At any time in the life of a paedophile that has already established a motivation to offend sexually towards a child, he may undergo one or more life experiences that can trigger a response invoking action of a sexually deviant nature – action such as masturbation while fantasising about sexually abusing a child.

Such experiences can be:

- depravation of sexual and/or emotional activity
- breakdown in emotional and sexual spousal/partner relationship
- stress/depression
- severe physical illness

- alcoholism
- drug dependency
- sudden exposure to abusive images of children – fuelling desire and being sexually stimulating
- sudden restriction of access to own or other's children – preventing the emotional expression/play/bonding that the paedophile has developed throughout his life (generally, or his preferred gender/age/descriptive type/range).

Like any other personally important and concerted acts carried out by humans, the physical sexual abuse of a child is considered and mapped out long before the event. The considerations given are vast, ranging from the sexual activity itself, planning, targeting an individual, overcoming internal and external inhibitors, and the grooming process. Throughout these stages, the paedophiles will fantasise, regularly, sometimes 20 to 30 times a day, or more.

Child abusive sexual fantasy plays a major part in the offending cycle and has two main areas of concern: firstly, that the fantasy is of sexual thought or desire towards a child and secondly, that the fantasised acts are illegal. People who have explored the nature of their sexual abuse of children will often refer to fantasy as the 'fuel for offending'. (Sullivan 2000/2001)

While fantasy about sexually abusing a child during masturbation is probably the primary fantasy, many paedophiles fantasise concerning the control, manipulation and suffering of the child victim and sometimes the victim's family. More importantly, fantasy, particularly to the point of orgasm, though diminishing the urge to offend directly post orgasm, leads to strengthen and reinforce the overall urge to gain contact with a child, control a child, justify the proposed illegal action of sexual abuse, and to ascend to physically sexually abusing the child.

Fantasy also allows the paedophile to rehearse every aspect of his planning, targeting, grooming and, finally, his physical sexual assault. He can play in his mind every detail just as he likes it, exactly to his choice and personal preference. His method of sexual abuse will know no boundaries, which is a fearsome prospect for a strong-minded, resolute, skilled and manipulative paedophiliac sexual offender who at this stage has the beginnings of the desire and willingness to undergo whatever it takes to overcome his feelings of guilt, anxiety and conscience.

Child abusive sexual fantasy can also generate emotion and sexual desire of sufficient magnitude that the paedophile is driven to a point where he is psychologically determined to overcome all obstacles that prevent or impede his abusive path. Having already overcome his 'internal inhibitors' at this stage of motivation, external inhibitors can now be confronted and are very often conquered.

Examples of *external inhibitors*:

- people who will safeguard the child and prevent easy access
- fear of being caught – by the authorities
- retribution – by victim, by victim's family, by the public
- exposure to the media

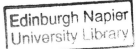

- imprisonment
- short- or long-term intrusive monitoring by police/probation/local authority
- loss of contact with or disownment by family members
- social ostracism
- possessing features and/or characteristics that are, in the general public's view, stereotypical to that of child molesters
- inability to form relationships and/or communicate easily and effectively with children or own peer groups, thereby appearing 'odd' or 'unusual' and thus creating an increased risk of having one's true intentions exposed.

Planning

For some paedophiles, the process of planning the sexual abuse of a child creates an intriguing, challenging and an enjoyable activity, which often stimulates the paedophile in both psychological and sexual desire. Masturbation often occurs at this stage, fantasising over the issue of gaining access, gaining control and the sexually abusive behaviour itself.

Planning will take into consideration many aspects such as making the initial contact with parents or carers, formulating a plausible subterfuge, isolating the child from parents or carers, exerting compelling and incomparable control over the chosen victim, continuing to 'keep the child quiet' and 'getting away with it'.

Throughout this process, the paedophile will be psychologically confronting the obvious and apparent external inhibitors. He will grow in confidence as he mentally 'plans' and 'manoeuvres' his way around them, fuelling his motivation and bringing him ever nearer to the point of offending.

Targets

The selection of an appropriate victim will depend primarily on availability, suitability and ability.

Availability to the paedophile

Paedophiles, like any other group of people, have sexual preferences although the strength of the preference will vary from one paedophile to another. For some, the need to engage sexually with the 'physically ideal' is so great that they will wait months or even years to successfully offend. For others, forgoing the 'physically ideal' is an acceptable loss in order to gain sexual gratification; on occasions, even transcending gender. Availability is also governed by aspects of the level of protection afforded to the child by the parents or carers.

Suitability

Suitability can be determined by a number of factors. These factors, either singularly or collectively, can, to the perceptive paedophile, announce a child's likelihood to be successfully 'groomed' – the most obvious factors being the amount of attention the child requires balanced against that which the child actually receives, appearance of vulnerability, the child's lack of maturity, low level of intellect for the child's age, the child's willingness to be led, being fearful of adults, possessing social ineptitude; and, most concerning, having a previous history of sexual abuse victimisation.

Ability

Seductive, prolonged continual sexual offending is greatly dependent upon the skill level and experience of the offender. Like any other complicated and in-depth activity, successful paedophiliac offending has to be learnt. Many initial 'trial-and-error' events take place, usually involving minor grooming practices and no physical offending. Practising, rehearsing and honing skills such as making contact with parents or carers, gaining access to children, blending into the background and grooming adults and children is paramount if the paedophile is to enjoy any future successful and unchallenged paedophiliac sexual activity.

Grooming

This is a recent term added to the English language that can be used to describe the manipulation and control of another – primarily children. Grooming can begin with the parents or carers of a child, it can involve just one person or it can involve a whole community. During the grooming process, the paedophile will continue to grow in confidence, combat external inhibitors and develop his skill base.

It is at this stage in the cycle that the most severe psychological damage to a child can be caused. Paedophiles will stop at nothing to gain control of a child and can use such measures as violence or the threat of violence against the child or a loved one, driving a wedge between child and parent, undermine the parents' love for the child, reduce the child's self-worth, use blackmail, bribery or corruption.

Throughout the period of grooming, the paedophile will again be masturbating while fantasising about his achievements and the developing prospect to fully sexually offend. Some paedophiles will constantly 'groom' (both adults and children). They will work continually, to gain trust and support from anyone, as they perceive this to assist them in the edification of themselves in the community and in gaining respect and acceptance. They will be constantly searching for opportunities to engage with parents and children, thereby widening the scope for future victims.

Masturbates to fantasy/rehearsal

The paedophile at this stage is in a position to seriously consider moving forward to physical offending. Virtually everything is in place and he is able to masturbate while rehearsing in his mind the actual sexual abuse that he is in a position to successfully carry out. At the same time, he masturbates and fantasises, probably almost continuously, about actions and deeds of which he is uncertain of success, but would like to attempt and achieve.

The paedophile's continual masturbation and fantasy also serves to reinforce his resolve concerning internal inhibitors. Very often, the 'way around' or to 'overcome' a stumbling block is to view the situation through 'distorted thinking' or 'cognitive distortion'. This is to re-invent any given situation or circumstance to fit one's own choosing and is not subject solely to sex offending. Many people, in many circumstances, cognitively distort the truth to make their action and continued action acceptable to themselves. For example, the smoker making a poor attempt to 'give up' may well distort the truth by telling himself '. . . one more won't hurt, no-one will find out and I can stop at any time . . .' Cognitive distortions lessen the blow, make the situation more agreeable, and create a belief in oneself that the illegal and immoral actions of child sexual abuse are acceptable and even appear justifiable.

Cognitive distortions (distorted thinking)

Distorted thinking has many forms and can cause the paedophile to feel fully justified and blameless for his past, current or intended paedophiliac behaviour and offences.

These are the most common forms of distorted thinking.

- Denial – as detailed above, this can be blatant; it can also be supported with elaborate stories of illness, misunderstanding, conspiracy or vengeance by another. In the right circumstances, the offender may well begin to believe his own lie, convincing himself of his innocence. The paedophile may also deny that the child has any sexually arousing effect on him – this denial could be to himself or to others.
- Minimisation – this is very often a distorted thought of the guilty sex offender. As an example, an adult male performing digital penetration on a four-year-old girl, either vaginally or anally, may well minimise his actions, describing what he has done as 'I just touched her – didn't really do any harm'.
- Normalisation – the belief that what the paedophile is thinking is in fact what everyone else is thinking. The paedophile firmly believes that he is acting normally and that anyone not thinking or acting the same way is the 'odd man out'.
- Justification – overtly demonstrates a lifestyle of correct behaviour to counter-balance allegations of abuse. He may well tell himself, as well as others, that he is a 'good man', an 'honest man', a man that regularly attends church, helps the needy, has helped the victim and the victim's family.
- Blame – places the responsibility for his sexual abuse upon the victim: '. . . she was asking me about sex so I showed her . . . he wanted to know what masturbation was, so I let him do it to me to teach him . . . she led me on, she knew what she was doing and seduced me . . . he kept on wanting to look at my porno mags, so I showed him them and one thing led to another . . .' or places the blame upon other people: '. . . my wife won't have sex with me any more and I found myself just doing it to this girl . . .'
- Excuses – 'I was drunk, I didn't know what I was doing . . . I was depressed about losing my job, I wasn't thinking straight . . . I haven't had sex in a while and she looked so good, I thought she was old enough . . . I was abused as a child and I thought it was an okay thing to do . . . I kept all the indecent photographs to avoid physically offending . . .'

- Assigns adult issues or motives onto children – distorting innocent conversation as a method of seduction.
- Presents the absence or failure of prosecution as evidence of innocence – a guilty paedophile who was not charged, or was acquitted due to a technicality, may well believe himself to be innocent and use the court's findings to support his claim of future innocence.
- Terminology – a paedophile may well use 'other' words or phrases to describe his victims or his behaviour. In the paedophile's eyes a boy or youth becomes a 'young man', a girl becomes a 'young lady'. The paedophile's sexual love of a particular child becomes 'I like the company of children'.

Commits assault

The initial or even sole assault may well be very minor; in fact maybe nothing more than an inappropriate, quick, brush-like touch, often outside of clothing, which the victim may fail to recognise as an indecent assault. Conversely, the weeks or months of planning, targeting and grooming may have resulted in the paedophile having a completely safe environment in which to offend; as well as 'building up' a heightened sexual desire and anticipation, after which the abuser attempts and/or carries out a severe assault involving either or both digital or penile penetration.

Masturbates

The paedophile will re-live the assault over and over again, masturbating to the recollection. If the assault was minor, masturbation may well serve to create a desire to commit further and more severe assaults, and also continue to reinforce the paedophile's belief (cognitive distortion) that what he is doing is not wrong, as perhaps no physical harm was caused.

If the assault was severe, masturbation may again serve to reinforce the paedophile's belief that what he is doing is not wrong as he may consider such factors as: no harm caused as no complaint made, the child liked it, again as no complaint has been made. Masturbation may also cause the paedophile to consider other physical acts to perform on the child victim, as he now feels confident that he can offend against his chosen victim whenever he chooses to do so.

Guilt relieved

Following the assault, the paedophile may experience feelings of guilt. Without a complaint made by the child victim or the victim's family, nothing really changes for the paedophile and so following continued masturbation, fantasy and cognitive distortion, the paedophile will push guilt away.

Pushes guilt away

The paedophile will distance himself from feelings of guilt in any number of ways, but primarily by cognitive distortion. He will lay blame for his actions on anyone but himself: '. . . my wife doesn't want sex so it's her fault for my having sex with our daughter . . . she was flaunting herself, so she obviously wanted to have sex with me – even though she is only nine, she knew what she was doing . . . he let me do it, he didn't object, he didn't cry out, so he must have liked and wanted to have sex with me . . .'

Guilt relieved

Having justified to himself that his illegal paedophiliac activities are in fact acceptable, feelings of guilt disappear.

Back to the beginning

Plans have been made and efficiently executed; internal and external inhibitors have been overcome; a target has been selected, groomed and successfully offended against; and guilt and victim sympathy has been rooted out by distorted thinking. All these factors bring the paedophile to the realisation that he has successfully, and without drawing attention to himself, sexually abused a child. These factors, combined with continual masturbation and fantasy, give rise to a powerful sexual desire and anticipation. He feels confident and motivated to 'do it again'. The paedophile is ready to continue in the cycle and to re-offend.

The following are extracts from an article based on a presentation given by Joe Sullivan MA (CRIM) BA (HONS) CQSW DIP PSY to the International Conference on Violence Towards Children, in Lisbon, Portugal, in February 2000 and repeated at a NOTA (National Organisation for the Treatment of Sex Offenders) conference workshop in September 2001.

Wolf and Eldridge – the cycle of sexual offending

Wolf's theory (1984) has been influential in shaping the understanding of sexual offending and illustrating the stages offenders will progress through in the lead up to and immediately following the abuse (*see* Figure 5.2). The model continues to be a central tenet of most common features of any offender's process of sexually abusing children. It is important for therapists not to attempt to make the offender fit the cycle but rather to use the framework as a means by which the offender can acknowledge the structure of his developing behaviour and explore it in detail.

Eldridge (1998) has developed the work of Wolf by introducing the concepts of the 'continuous cycle', the 'inhibited cycle' and the 'short-circuit cycle'. These cycles focus on the particular route an offender will take after the commission of the offence.

In the case of the continuous cycle, offenders will re-trace each of the stages of the cycle, selecting a new victim each time. This is perhaps the most common in the case of an offender with an indecent exposure pattern, where, having sexually offended, he will repeat the pattern in its entirety.

In the case of the inhibited cycle, the offender becomes blocked or inhibited following the commission of an offence and may stop for a period of time.

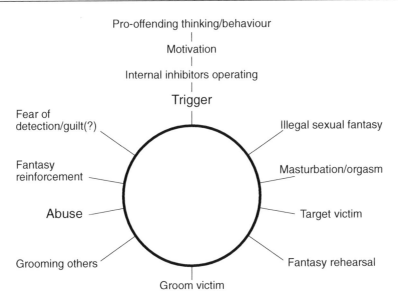

Figure 5.2   The cycle of offending (source: Wolf 1984).

In time, the offender finds a way to overcome these inhibitors and progress through the various stages of his cycle in order to commit another offence. Typically, this cycle relates to an offender who selects a new victim each time he offends, where he returns to general illegal sexual fantasy before choosing the next victim.

In the short-circuit cycle, the offender does not become inhibited following the

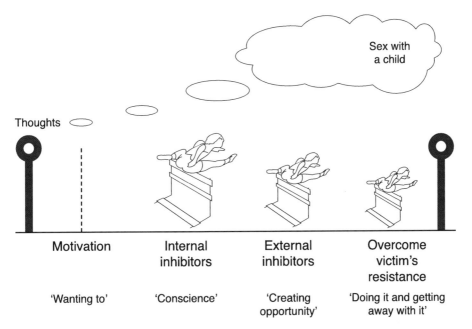

Figure 5.3   The four preconditions of sexual offending (source: Finkelhor 1986).

commission of the offence, but rather returns to the cycle at the point of fantasy rehearsal and speeds up. In this case, the offender continues to abuse either the same child or another in a similar manner. This cycle is typical where the offender is abusing a child in the family or within a context where he will have contact with the child.

Finkelhor – the four preconditions of sexual offending

Finkelhor (1984, 1986) has explored the motivations of offenders for engaging in sexual abuse and suggested four preconditions to sexual offending. Practitioners and clinicians have sought to illustrate this theory in a variety of ways. One method is to describe the preconditions as hurdles on a racecourse. Motivation to sexually offend would be the starting line. Internal inhibitors, external inhibitors and victim resistance would be the three hurdles, which an individual must negotiate in order to sexually offend. Figure 5.3 illustrates this clinical application of Finkelhor's four preconditions to sexual offending.

References

Eldridge H. *Therapist Guide for Maintaining Change: Relapse prevention for adult perpetrators of child sexual abuse*. Thousand Oaks, CA: Sage; 1998.
Finkelhor D. *Child Sexual Abuse: New theory and research*. London, Macmillan; 1984.
Finkelhor D. *A Sourcebook on Child Sexual Abuse*. Thousand Oaks, CA: Sage; 1986.
Sullivan J. Article based on a presentation to the International Conference on Violence Towards Children, Lisbon, Portugal; February 2000; repeated at a NOTA (National Organisation for the Treatment of Sex Offenders) conference workshop in September 2001.
Wolf SC. *A Multifactorial Model of Deviant Sexuality*. A paper presented at the Third International Conference of Victimology, Lisbon, Portugal; 1984.

Section One conclusion

Some adults possess a sexual and sometimes emotional interest in children. The interest can be heterosexual, homosexual or bisexual, and is defined as either paedophiliac, hebephiliac or both. Generally, such persons are referred to in our society solely as 'paedophiles'. Paedophilia and hebephilia are human sexual orientations, neither of which is a disease nor an illness which is open to cure. Therefore, the arousal of a paedophile's or hebephile's emotional and sexual desire, in conjunction with any ensuing illegal sexualised behaviour, can only be controlled. Such control will be generated by the influence imposed by either or both internal or external inhibitors. However, inhibitors can be overcome and, for most paedophiles and hebephiles, such inhibitors eventually are. Inhibitors are conquered by way of careful planning, strategic grooming and powerful cognitive distortions or 'distorted thinking'. In addition, a targeting paedophile or hebephile, possessing the propensity and susceptibility to offend, is substantially aided in his quest by parents and carers who choose to ignore the possibility of child sexual abuse occurring within their family unit. Parents who make such a perilous decision are very likely to fail in either observing or distinguishing recognisable characteristics and behavioural patterns which are common features of predatory paedophiles and hebephiles.

Children who are physically or mentally disabled are most at risk from sexual abusers. However, almost equally, children who are deprived of love and attention, who are spurned or made to feel of little value or have little self-worth may unwittingly present themselves as vulnerable targets.

Contrary to common belief, not all paedophiles and hebephiles are men. It is widely recognised that approximately 5% of adults who successfully sexually offend against children are women.

All paedophiliac and hebephiliac offenders possess recognisable characteristics and behavioural patterns which, when monitored and recorded, can lead to them being exposed as being the people most likely to pose a significant risk of sexual harm to children.

The degree of success experienced by a paedophile or a hebephile during his period of sexual abuse activity will largely depend upon the level of secrecy and security that is maintained. To achieve a high level of secrecy and security, grooming practices will include methods of 'keeping the child from telling'. These methods will vary from one offender to another, but will essentially involve blackmail, threats and instilling extreme fear into the mind of the chosen victim. In the vast majority of these cases, the victim will be exceptionally compliant and obedient, thus giving the offender complete and over-riding control, both at the time of the abuse and for many years thereafter.

Most offending paedophiles and hebephiles will not commit just one offence. Though some will offend every few months or every few years, the majority will offend or at least attempt to offend continuously. Most, if not all, will wilfully or subconsciously plan, select, target, fantasise, groom and finally sexually abuse a child; only to repeat the whole process in what is recognised as the 'cycle of offending'. This cycle is repeated time and time again throughout the offender's life and can only be broken by either the offender himself having the motivation to change or by exclusion from society, namely lifelong imprisonment.

Issues for parents to consider

Many parents refuse to accept that child sexual abuse could possibly occur within their immediate family unit. For fathers, this may be a 'macho-protector' ideology, but it is a dangerous ideology to harbour. Ignoring the possibility that sexual abuse could occur in one's own family is denying oneself the opportunity to identify the simplest of clues that may indicate your child has been targeted and is being groomed for sexual exploitation. As parents or carers, you must be prepared to accept the unacceptable, believe the unbelievable and prepare yourself as best you can to protect your child and prevent sexual abuse.

Consider what you ask or allow your child to do that may make him or her more vulnerable to a predatory paedophile, taking into consideration 'the selection of victims' as outlined in Chapter 3. Simply asking your child to regularly walk to the shops alone, albeit only a few yards, or wait alone at the corner of the street for the school bus may allow a paedophile to enforce his presence on your child and begin the grooming process. Also, consider what action you would take if you found your child to be in receipt of gifts from either a person unknown to you or a friend. If gifts are repeatedly given, and this continues to go unchallenged, your child may well believe that you consent to such 'gift-giving' and he or she will not refuse or challenge any future act or behaviour proposed by the paedophile.

Consider also 'the man next door', who is married with two children and has been known to you for many years. If he asks to borrow your nice new car for a few hours, the likelihood is you will say no. You may say yes, but this is likely to be with reservation. You are likely to be very worried and concerned, until the vehicle is returned and you are able to check for any damage. However, should the same married man ask if he could take your child on a day trip with his family you may feel, because he is married and has children of his own, that your child will be safe and therefore harbour little or no concern regarding child abuse issues. The male neighbour may be of no threat in any way to his own children but quite possibly, without his partner's knowledge, pose an immense risk of sexual harm to your child.

Consider how you may be allowing yourself to be influenced or guided by others. For example, the fact that a large number of responsible and caring parents from your local school choose to have their children educated by a private music teacher at his home address or private studio does not guarantee that the music teacher in question has been vetted by the police or the local authority. Nor does it mean that he has been recommended by the school or is indeed qualified. More significantly, being popular and well patronised is not an assurance that the teacher doesn't pose a significant risk of sexual or other abusive harm to your child. Your child could be the one child, out of 25 students he teaches, that he desires, targets and will groom for eventual sexual abuse.

Whatever the situation or circumstance, parents, carers and guardians need to take full responsibility for the safety of any child who is in their care.

Section Two

Recognising symptoms of child abuse

6

Recognisable signs of a child suffering emotional abuse

What is emotional child abuse?

By definition it is:

Emotional *adj* readily affected by or appealing to the emotions.
Abuse *v* use wrongly; ill-treat violently.

In 1999 the Department of Health produced a guide entitled *Working Together to Safeguard Children – a guide to inter-agency working to safeguard and promote the welfare of children*; the guide was revised in 2006. All the following relevant references are taken from the revised edition.

In the Department's guide, the term emotional abuse is described as follows:

Emotional abuse is the persistent emotional maltreatment of a child such as to cause severe and persistent adverse effects on a child's emotional development. It may involve conveying to a child that they are worthless or unloved, inadequate, or valued only insofar as they meet the needs of another person. It may feature age or developmentally inappropriate expectations being imposed on children. These may include interactions that are beyond the child's developmental capability, as well as overprotection and limitation of exploration and learning, or preventing the child participating in normal social interaction. It may involve seeing or hearing the ill-treatment of another. It may involve serious bullying causing children frequently to feel frightened or in danger, or the exploitation or corruption of children. Some level of emotional abuse is involved in all types of maltreatment of a child, though it may occur alone. (Department of Health 2006)

Such ill treatment can consist of one or more of the following deliberate acts:

- total rejection of a child – ignoring or having no regard for the child and affording the child little or no affection
- failing to communicate in any fashion with the child
- telling the child that he or she is not loved, is unwanted and having him or her in the first place was a mistake
- humiliating and ridiculing the child both in isolation and before other people; in particular, peer groups
- continually exposing a child to activities engineered for adults or adolescents of an older age, e.g. frightening funfair rides, horror films, specific flumes at water parks and fearsome adult computer games

- telling the child that he or she is worthless, again in isolation or in front of other people; in particular their peer group
- forcing a child to put the needs of parents or other family members before their own
- continual criticism of what the child does
- singling the child out within the family and telling them that they are less important than other children within the family group
- convincing the child that they are intellectually, educationally, socially or physically inadequate
- continual verbal abuse
- causing the child to believe that they are inferior to their peers
- threatening the child and laying blame on the child for the misbehaviour of other children
- causing the child to constantly feel frightened or in danger of harm.

The Department of Health's guide continues, outlining the possible impact of emotional abuse:

> There is increasing evidence of the adverse long-term consequences for children's development where they have been subject to sustained emotional abuse, including the impact of serious bullying. Emotional abuse has an important impact on a developing child's mental health, behaviour and self-esteem. It can be especially damaging in infancy. Underlying emotional abuse may be as important, if not more so, than other more visible forms of abuse in terms of its impact on the child. Domestic violence is abusive in itself. Adult mental health problems and parental substance misuse may be features in families where children are exposed to such abuse. (Department of Health 2006)

A child suffering emotional abuse may display any one of the following symptoms

Being withdrawn, appearing isolated and lonely, failing to interact with peers

The child may choose not to speak very much, may be reluctant to join in games or songs and generally refrain from becoming involved with adults or children. They may sit alone very quietly, keeping themselves to themselves.

Poor performance at school and truanting

The influence of emotional abuse may well cause the child to perform poorly in schoolwork. Education and learning expectations placed upon children by teachers and parents are added pressures that the child at this point does not want. They may well find escaping from school a short-term relief. Truanting also prevents the child having to face other children who may tease and taunt them about their timidity and/or isolation.

The child's stress, worry and upset, added to his or her inability to interact with others or concentrate, may well cause the child to be slow in learning and fall behind with their studies, giving a false representation of their true intellectual level.

Tantrums and behaviour inconsistent with child's age

If challenged on difficult matters, the child may throw a tantrum. This is not uncommon for younger children, but children of 10 or 11 years of age have generally outgrown this behaviour. If a child of 10 or 11 years is regularly throwing tantrums, consideration should be given to the possibility that the behaviour is a symptom of emotional abuse.

Other age-regressed behaviour could also identify emotional abuse, such as thumb sucking, talking in a manner suited to a younger child or playing with toys usually associated with younger children.

Maturity regression, wishes to be treated as a younger child

A child suffering emotional abuse may well want to be treated as a child much younger than their psychological years. This may include baby talk, being fed by an adult, carried or cuddled like a younger child, not wanting to interact with children of their own age and appearing much happier playing with younger children and their toys.

Attention seeking

This type of behaviour can occur within the home towards a parent or guardian, or in school towards staff or other children, or in any public arena where adults or children are in view.

The attention-seeking behaviour can consist of any one of the following:

- continual naughtiness
- continual crying or whining
- persistent wetting or soiling of clothes or bed
- being physically abusive towards other children or adults
- running away from home or school
- deliberately damaging toys or property.

Aggressive behaviour

'The best form of defence is attack.' An emotionally abused child, who is frightened of other children and/or adults, may well protect his or her fear by overzealously threatening or attacking others. The aggressive behaviour may not be initially obvious; it may manifest through sporting games or general play.

Failure to develop and thrive, eating and sleeping disorders

Many emotionally abused children fail to develop and thrive as expected, both physically and psychologically. Physical underdevelopment can be as a result of not eating and/or not digesting correctly. This does not mean that the child is being ill-fed or starved, but that emotional upset is causing them to be 'off' their food. This can result in weight loss and a failure to grow, causing them to look thin, gaunt and small for their age.

Insufficient teaching of basic skills by a parent can lead a child to be psychologically underdeveloped. Almost from the moment of birth, mental stimulus and education, particularly in aspects of personal behaviour, are vital for a child; failing to understand or be competent in basic skills can be detrimental to learning abilities in later years.

Emotional worry, fear or stress may well disrupt the child's sleep. The child may appear continually tired, listless and drawn, and be slow in responding to mental or physical stimulation.

Loss of confidence coupled with low self-esteem

The child may lack confidence and require a great deal of coaxing to become engaged in, and complete, the most simplistic of tasks. If confident enough to speak, they may well inform carers that they feel unable to accomplish anything. They may feel generally inadequate.

Self-neglect

Children may fail to care for themselves. This is not unusual for a young child, but most 10 to 12 year olds and teenagers, particularly girls, care about their appearance, wearing the latest fashions and wanting to be attractive to the opposite sex. A child suffering from emotional abuse may have little thought concerning their own appearance.

Self-harm

Children suffering emotional abuse, as with any other abuse, may physically harm themselves. The self-harm may take many forms such as cutting of flesh, particularly their arms, wrists and hands. They may also cut their hair. Sometimes they may cut themselves on areas of the body which are not commonly visible, such as the upper arms, chest and thighs.

Drug and alcohol abuse

As a means of escape, a child suffering emotional abuse may well succumb to the taking of alcohol or other drugs such as cannabis, heroin or crack cocaine. This can also be a method of self-harm.

Child is wary of their parents and other adults, and may cling to one particular adult

The child may show distrust of male and/or female adults. If they fear their parents, the child may well identify another adult, possibly a teacher or childminder, with whom they find refuge and security. The child may become extremely emotionally attached to this adult and display these feelings by physically clinging to them whenever possible. The child will demonstrate quite vividly the desire of not wanting to let go.

Associated mental illnesses (psychosomatic)

A child may display signs of an illness that cannot be explained, known as a psychosomatic illness. This is caused by the child's mental or emotional state rather than any physical factors.

Note

It must be recognised that a child may display any one or more of the above symptoms and not be experiencing emotional abuse. There may be other reasons such as sexual abuse, physical abuse or bullying, etc. A child acting with one of the above symptoms should alert you to the fact that the child is suffering in some way. A child acting with a number of the above symptoms indicates probable emotional abuse.

Reference

Department of Health. *Working Together to Safeguard Children – a guide to inter-agency working to safeguard and promote the welfare of children*. London: Department of Health; 2006. http://www.everychildmatters.gov.uk/resources-and-practice/IG00060

7

Recognisable signs of a child suffering physical abuse

What is physical child abuse?

By definition it is:

Physical   *adj*   of the body; as contrasted with the mind or spirit.
Abuse   *v*   use wrongly; ill-treat violently.

In 1999 the Department of Health produced a guide entitled *Working Together to Safeguard Children – a guide to inter-agency working to safeguard and promote the welfare of children*; the guide was revised in 2006. All the following relevant references are taken from the revised edition.

In the Department's guide, the term physical abuse is described as follows:

Physical abuse may involve hitting, shaking, throwing, poisoning, burning or scalding, drowning, suffocating or otherwise causing physical harm to a child. Physical harm may also be caused when a parent or carer fabricates the symptoms of, or deliberately induces, illness in a child. (Department of Health 2006)

Physical abuse of a child may also occur when an adult or other child inflicts on a child any one or more of the following additional deliberate physical acts:

* cutting of flesh or stabbing
* pinching, twisting or squeezing any part of the child's body
* punching or beating the child with the hands
* beating the child with an instrument (belt or stick)
* throwing a child to the floor or other surface
* kicking
* forcing the child to stand or sit either in an unbearable position, or on a surface which causes pain, for a prolonged period
* making the child remain in an overly hot or overly cold environment, sometimes with inappropriate clothing.

Fabricated or Induced Illnesses by Carers (Munchausen syndrome/ Munchausen syndrome by proxy)

In February 2002, the Working Party of the Royal College of Paediatrics and Child Health produced a report outlining issues concerning Fabricated or Induced

Illnesses (FII) by Carers and Munchausen syndrome. The report accepted the views of R Meadow, in that four main issues exist:

1 Illness in a child which is fabricated or induced by a parent or a person who is in *loco parentis.*
2 A child is presented for medical assessment and care, usually persistently, often resulting in multiple medical procedures.
3 The perpetrator denies the aetiology of the illness.
4 Acute symptoms and signs cease when the child is separated from the perpetrator.

It must be noted that points 3 and 4 are often relevant in many child abuse cases. The report also agreed with the findings of Fisher *et al.* (1995) in that

The condition known as Munchausen Syndrome by Proxy or other variations does not satisfy criteria for acceptance as a discrete medical syndrome because of the wide variation. (Working Party of the Royal College of Paediatrics and Child Health 2002)

The report continues:

Semantically the term Munchausen Syndrome by Proxy is only valid when a person who has Munchausen Syndrome themselves uses others, particularly children, to manifest their disorder. We should note that even when one parent has Munchausen Syndrome it may be the other parent who is harming the child. We must not be diverted by arguments over semantics. Fabrication or illness induction include all forms of such activity and do not inevitably clarify the motivation of the carer, which may be difficult to ascertain. It can include the old terms MSbP (Munchausen Syndrome by Proxy) or MbPS (Munchausen by Proxy Syndrome) whether applied to the carer, child or scenario, and includes delusion, excessive anxiety, masquerade, hysteria, doctor shopping, doctor addiction, mothering to death, seekers of personal help or attention or financial gain, and those who fail to give needed treatment as well as those who treat unnecessarily. (Working Party of the Royal College of Paediatrics and Child Health 2002)

The report recommends that paediatricians use the term Fabricated or Induced Illnesses.

Impact of physical abuse

The Department of Health's guide continues, outlining the possible impact of physical abuse:

Physical abuse can lead directly to neurological damage, physical injuries, disability or – at extreme – death. Harm may be caused to children both by the abuse itself, and by the abuse taking place in a wider family or institutional context of conflict and aggression, including inappropriate or inexpert use of physical restraint. Physical abuse has been linked to aggressive behaviour in children, emotional and behavioural problems, and educational difficulties. Violence is pervasive and the physical abuse of children frequently coexists with domestic violence. (Department of Health 2006)

A child suffering physical abuse may display any one of the following

Bruising

Signs of bruising on an immobile child (baby)

It is very unlikely that a baby, yet to become mobile (crawling or walking), will bruise itself.

Bruises of various shapes

Bruising in the shape of fingers or of a flat hand on one part of the body, arms or legs indicates that the child has been struck. Similar bruising encircling the body, arms or legs indicates the child has been grabbed or gripped tightly. If the bruising is in the shape of two hands, encircling the sides of the abdomen, it is a possibility that the child has been held tightly and possibly shaken.

Bruises overlapping others and of different colours

Bruises vary in colour depending on the severity of the injury and the duration for which the body's self-healing process has had the opportunity to work. If bruises of different colours appear in the same area of a child's body and appear to be overlapping each other, it is likely that the child is suffering repeated physical abuse.

Facial bruising

Bruising to the face, particularly the cheeks, is often caused by the parent or guardian following periods of frustration or stress. It often arises when the child will not feed and the parent or guardian attempts to force-feed the child, and tightly grips the child's head. When this occurs with babies, evidence of a ruptured fraenulum (a small membrane lying between the inside of the upper lip and upper jaw) is often found.

Black eyes

On babies (immobile) black eyes will be as a result of physical abuse.

On babies (mobile) and young children, black eyes are commonly caused through physical abuse. A child crawling or walking into a wall, door or cupboard, or tripping and falling onto a flat surface, is likely to cause bruising about his or her forehead, nose or chin. Black eyes are caused usually by direct blows to the eye socket area with a clenched fist, or thumbs pushing directly against the eyeball.

Burns

In most common domestic environments, a burn will be one of two types, either a scald or a contact burn.

Scalds, accidental or deliberate, occur when a liquid of a sufficient temperature comes into contact with the skin for an adequate period of time to damage the surface and underlying layers of skin and flesh. In most cases of scalding, the liquid concerned is hot water – either tap water, boiling water or a hot drink. Other liquids which may cause scalding can be soup, molten foodstuffs such as chocolate or sugar, molten metal such as solder, oil or grease, or candle wax.

Contact burns – accidental or deliberate – usually occur when an implement at a sufficient temperature comes into contact with skin, again for an adequate period of time to damage the surface and underlying layers of skin and flesh. Most contact burns can be considered to be 'brand-like', in that the burn replicates the size and shape of the implement. Common contact-burn implements are cigarettes, matches, cigarette lighters, steam irons, cooking hobs, soldering irons, fireside tools such as tongs or pokers, or hair curlers.

Unlikely site of a burn or scald

Burns and scalds on the child's body in unlikely places are usually the result of physical abuse. The chosen locations will be areas where the injury is less likely to be noticed by teachers, carers or visitors. The most common areas for such injuries are:

- under the arms
- on the inside of the mouth
- on the soles of the feet
- in or around the anus
- in or around the vagina
- or any location where the injury would normally be hidden by clothing or out of sight unless medically examined.

Accidental burning or scalding usually results in a mark that is irregular in shape and without definition, e.g. a splash of boiling water making contact with the skin, or a tip of a finger touching a hot surface.

A malicious scald is more likely to be a regular shape and well defined, e.g. a hand deliberately held in a cup of boiling water will show a defined mark about the wrist or forearm, often giving the injured hand the visual impression of a glove. Similarly, a foot and lower leg deliberately immersed in saucepan of boiling water will often give the visual appearance of a stocking or sock clad leg.

A malicious contact burn, caused by placing a hot poker against the under-arm, will clearly define the shape of the poker and any markings upon it.

Cigarette burns

Circular burn marks, approximately 8–10 mm in diameter, are likely to be the result of physical abuse. Most malicious cigarette burns are caused by the abuser bringing the lighted cigarette into contact with the skin at a right angle (90 degrees); this produces a neat circle. Malicious cigarette burns are also likely to cut deeply into the skin. It is usual for an abuser to burn a child with a cigarette on many occasions, leaving evidence of multiple burn injuries.

Accidental cigarette burns are usually an irregular shape and mark the skin lightly. This is due to the cigarette being brought into contact with the skin at an odd angle, with little pressure and only for a brief moment.

Bites and fingernail injuries

Bites

The parts of a child's body that are the easiest to bite and the most commonly bitten are the hands, forearms, legs and feet, ears, nose and mouth. However, the abuser, if acting with self-protective thought, may attempt to hide the injury and bite on the less visible parts of the body, such as the insides of the thighs, the inner upper arms or in the centre of the buttocks. Bites to the hands, arms and possibly face can be the result of another child's violent behaviour; however, a medical practitioner can differentiate between evidence of an adult's bite and that of a child.

Fingernail injuries

In addition to bruising by gripping hard, the abuser may go on to digging his or her fingernails into the flesh of the child. Again these are common on arms and hands, but can also appear about the mouth and face if a child is not feeding well and force is used to open the mouth.

Broken bones and internal injuries

Broken bones

Some bones can be broken without any external evidence of injury. A child suffering with such an injury may be able to walk, stand or sit, but may do so awkwardly or with difficulty. Similarly, a child's unnoticed broken limb may be carried in an unusual position or move in an unnatural fashion. A child with a broken bone may walk and stand without an obvious display of injury or pain, but is unlikely to be able to sit without showing signs of discomfort.

Internal injuries

An internal injury, i.e. damage to kidneys, liver, lungs, intestine, etc., may cause any one of the following:

- vomiting food
- vomiting blood
- breathing difficulties
- fever and/or intense pain.

Head injuries

Blow to cranium

In simplistic terms, the human brain is suspended within the cranium by fluid and thin membranes. If the head suffers a violent jerk, the brain can collide with the lining of the skull causing bruising and damage to the brain. A blow to any part of the cranium can cause such a collision, as can violent shaking of a child. A blow to the head may cause a surface injury but this may not be visible as it may be hidden beneath the hair.

Whether the cranium is fractured or not, a blow may cause any of the following:

- vomiting food
- feeling nauseous, drowsiness, fitting, fainting, lack of concentration and a failure to interact as normal
- the child may look ill, appearing drawn, tired, and lethargic
- skin may appear either pale or red/purple in colour.

Shaking

Violent shaking of a child, of any age, can cause the brain to collide with the lining of the skull and therefore cause any of the above.

In addition, shaking can cause severe damage to the thin membranes which lie between the brain and the lining of the skull. If this occurs, it is very likely that the resulting bleeding will form blood clots, causing brain damage and, in some cases, lead to death.

> Physical abuse can be suspected and identified on occasions, not as a direct result of finding an injury, but by the actions and general behaviour of the parents or carers at the time of the finding, and the circumstances surrounding the cause of the injury. Suspicions can be raised by any of the following.

History of child physical abuse within the family group or known carers, or the child is a previous victim

Obviously, if a child or children within a certain family group are repeatedly presented to the authorities or medical practitioners with physical injuries, which by their nature alone raise concerns, then the sustaining of further injuries should at least give grounds for greater concern and call for the cause to be thoroughly investigated.

Inconsistent or vague account by the child as to the cause of injury, or the explanation appears practised, as if instructed

A child who has been deliberately injured by an adult or older child may be forced, by fear or threat, to give a spurious account as to the cause of the injury.

The child, if in pain or dazed for example, may forget the tale and give a true or another spurious account, which will conflict with that given by the culprit or person protecting the culprit.

The child appears uncomfortable or frightened when questioned regarding the cause of the injury

Again, through fear or threat, a deliberately injured child may be influenced to give a false account as to the cause of injury and fail to respond in a typical fashion when questioned. The degree of fear that is felt or how uncomfortable the child appears may vary if the person inducing the fear is present at the time when the child is questioned.

The abuser's explanation of the injuries is unrealistic

As written in 'Black eyes' above, an explanation for a child's injury may not tally with the physical injury that the child displays.
Examples:

1   A child with perfectly formed circular red marks measuring 8–10 mm in diameter, dotted across its back, has not been subjected to an accidental brush against a lit cigarette.
2   A non-mobile, four-month-old baby will not suffer an accidental black eye, or ruptured fraenulum, or repeated bruising to the face by its own actions of striking itself with its own hands and arms, or moving against the side of the cot, or dropping a suitable toy upon itself.
3   A baby or young child will not suffer a scald to the hand that has a clear and neat edge (suggesting the hand has been held in boiling water) if boiling water accidentally splashes on the child's hand.
4   A baby or young child will not suffer accidental brain damage or even death as a result of a minor or gentle shake.

Injuries occurring only when the child has specific changes in routine

Regular visits to the child's estranged father, or visits to the family group by an uncle, or school holidays spent with grandmother are all occasions when the child is out of routine. Should injuries occur during these time periods, or conversely out of these time periods, the persons responsible for the injuries can be clearly suspected and investigations should be put underway.

Severe injuries that have not received medical treatment

Should an abuser cause an obviously deliberate, serious or major injury to child, it is highly unlikely that the abuser will happily allow the child to be examined by a medical practitioner. Untreated deep burns or severe scalds are easy to recognise, as these may be wounds that are weeping, open, peeling and very painful.

Untreated broken bones and internal injuries are less obviously recognised. It is only at a later stage, perhaps when the child is being medically examined months or even years later, that self-healed injuries displaying poorly fused bones or internal scarring, etc., are identified.

Child constantly or routinely being kept at home and not attending school

Parents or carers who are responsible for deliberately inflicting physical injuries upon their children may well attempt to hide the visible evidence. This may

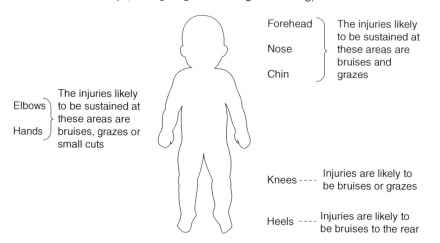

Figure 7.1   Common areas of skin or bone damage on a baby – consistent with accidental injury.

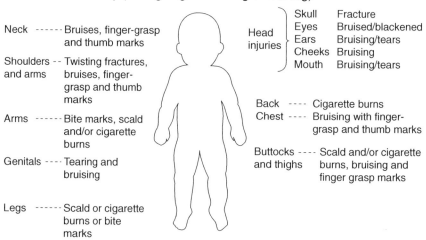

Figure 7.2   Common areas of skin or bone damage on a baby – consistent with non-accidental injury.

include not allowing their children (while the visible evidence is present) to attend school or go out to play with other children.

Possible resulting behaviour displayed by child suffering physical abuse

In addition to displaying the injuries as described above, a physically abused child may demonstrate one or more of the behaviours described below:

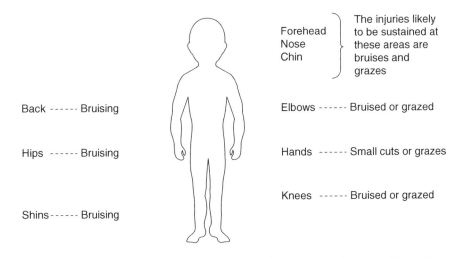

Forehead
Nose
Chin
}
The injuries likely to be sustained at these areas are bruises and grazes

Back ------ Bruising

Hips ------ Bruising

Shins ------ Bruising

Elbows ------ Bruised or grazed

Hands ------ Small cuts or grazes

Knees ------ Bruised or grazed

Figure 7.3 Common areas of skin or bone damage consistent with accidental injury.

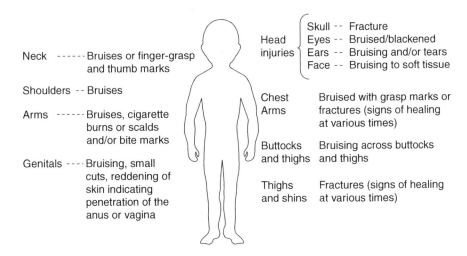

Head injuries
{
Skull -- Fracture
Eyes -- Bruised/blackened
Ears -- Bruising and/or tears
Face -- Bruising to soft tissue
}

Neck ------ Bruises or finger-grasp and thumb marks

Shoulders -- Bruises

Arms ------ Bruises, cigarette burns or scalds and/or bite marks

Genitals ---- Bruising, small cuts, reddening of skin indicating penetration of the anus or vagina

Chest Arms   Bruised with grasp marks or fractures (signs of healing at various times)

Buttocks and thighs   Bruising across buttocks and thighs

Thighs and shins   Fractures (signs of healing at various times)

Figure 7.4 Common areas of skin or bone damage consistent with non-accidental injury.

- constantly exhibits low self-esteem
- always presents him or herself as being keen to please
- avoids contact with peers whenever able
- shows extreme concern and anxiety about being reprimanded
- fails to display any feelings or emotions – never becomes excited, never exhibits an appearance of sadness, facial expression simply remains 'blank'
- fails to maintain a concentration span which is consistent with child's age and mental development
- shows little interest in hygiene or personal presentation
- may well act in a restless or even a hyperactive fashion.

See Figures 7.1 to 7.4 for common areas of skin or bone damage consistent with accidental and non-accidental injury.

References

Department of Health. *Working Together to Safeguard Children – a guide to inter-agency working to safeguard and promote the welfare of children.* London: Department of Health; 2006. http://www.everychildmatters.gov.uk/resources-and-practice/IG00060

Fisher GC, Mitchell I *et al*. Is Munchausen syndrome by proxy really a syndrome? *Arch Dis Child*. 72: 534–8; 1995.

Working Party of the Royal College of Paediatrics and Child Health. *Fabricated or Induced Illness by Carers*. 2002. www.rcpch.ac.uk/publications/recent_publications/FII.pdf

8

Recognisable signs of a child suffering sexual abuse

What is sexual child abuse?

By definition it is:

Sexual *adj* sexual feelings or behaviour; sexually exciting or attractive.
Abuse *v* use wrongly; ill-treat violently.

In 1999 the Department of Health produced a guide entitled *Working Together to Safeguard Children – a guide to inter-agency working to safeguard and promote the welfare of children*; the guide was revised in 2006. All the following relevant references are taken from the revised edition.

In the Department's guide, the term sexual abuse is described as follows:

Sexual abuse involves forcing or enticing a child or young person to take part in sexual activities, including prostitution, whether or not the child is aware of what is happening. The activities may involve physical contact, including penetrative (e.g. rape or buggery or oral sex) or non-penetrative acts. They may include non-contact activities, such as involving children in looking at, or in the production of, photographic material or watching sexual activities or encouraging children to behave in sexually inappropriate ways. (Department of Health 2006)

Based on work completed by Schechter and Roberge (1976), Kempe and Kempe (1978) define child sexual abuse as:

The involvement of dependent, developmentally immature children and adolescents in sexual activities which they do not fully comprehend, are unable to give informed consent to and that violate social taboos of family roles. (Kempe and Kempe 1978)

Angus and Woodward later defined child sexual abuse as:

Sexual abuse is any act which exposes a child to, or involves a child in, sexual processes beyond his or her understanding or contrary to accepted community standards. (Angus and Woodward 1995)

In more detailed terms, sexual abuse of a child occurs when an adult, or other child, uses a child for sexual gratification by way of inflicting upon a child, or causing a child to perform, any one or more of the following deliberate sexually motivated acts:

- sexual intercourse, both vaginal and anal, even if child appears to be a willing participant (unlawful sexual intercourse or sexual assault upon a child by penetration); this also includes an adult female having sexual intercourse with a male child
- sexual intercourse, both vaginal and anal, against child's will (rape)
- digital penetration (fingers) of vagina and/or anus
- inserting objects into a child's vagina, mouth or anus for sexual gratification
- adult, or other child, forcing child to perform oral sex
- adult, or other child, performing oral sex on child
- caressing or fondling child, particularly about the genital and/or breast area, in a sexualised fashion
- forcing a child to caress or fondle the genitals of another (adult or child)
- kissing and cuddling of child for sexual gratification (offender later fantasises about child he has cuddled)
- forcing child to perform sex acts with others for payment or reward
- exposing child to adult pornography in an attempt to seduce child and/or reduce child's sexual inhibitions
- exposing child to indecent images of children (children interacting with adults and/or other children) so as to convince child that sex between children and adults/children is normal and acceptable
- photographing a child in sexual poses
- adult exposing genitals (no physical contact) to child
- purposefully, for sexual gratification, observing a child undress, take a bath or utilise a toilet.

The Home Office's *Working Together to Safeguard Children* continues, outlining the possible impact of sexual abuse:

Disturbed behaviour including self-harm, inappropriate sexualised behaviour, depression and loss of self-esteem, have all been linked to sexual abuse. Its adverse effects may endure into adulthood. The severity of impact on a child is believed to increase the longer abuse continues, the more extensive the abuse, and the older the child. A number of features of sexual abuse have also been linked with severity of impact, including the relationship of the abuser to the child, the extent of premeditation, the degree of threat or coercion, sadism, and bizarre or unusual elements. A child's ability to cope with the experience of sexual abuse, once recognised or disclosed, is strengthened by the support of a non-abusive adult carer who believes the child, helps the child understand the abuse, and is able to offer help and protection. The reactions of practitioners also have an impact on the child's ability to cope with what has happened, and his or her feelings of self worth.

A proportion of adults who sexually abuse children have themselves been sexually abused as children. They may also have been exposed as children to domestic violence and discontinuity of care. However, it would be quite wrong to suggest that most children who are abused will inevitably go on to become abusers themselves. (Department of Health 2006)

> **Note**
> In many child sexual abuse cases, where sexual intercourse has taken place, the abusers have claimed that the child was a willing participant, or that they had 'informed consent' from the child. It must be recognised that children cannot give lawful consent for sexual intercourse until they reach the age of 16 (*see* Chapter 1, 'Understanding sexual orientation and paedophilia'). In many cases, the child may appear to give consent, by way of not refusing to engage in sexual activity or allowing sexual activity to commence. In many such cases, the child is often too heavily influenced by the abuser to resist or refuse the abuser's sexual advances; usually due to imposed fear or reward; most commonly, the controlling influence is fear.

The induced fear may vary in its form; it may result from the threat of physical harm or not wanting to get the abuser into trouble (this is very often the case when the abuser is the child's father or stepfather). The fear may also stem from not wishing to risk breaking up or damaging the family group.

If the child is very young and has been led to believe by the abuser that the continued sexual activity between them is normal and most 'daddies' or 'friends' act this way, then the child may not understand that what is occurring is wrong and therefore not make any attempt to refuse.

A child suffering sexual abuse may display any one of the following

Physical signs and symptoms

Injuries

A child, having suffered sexual abuse, may display any one of the following injuries:

- swelling, bruising or reddening of the skin or grazes, cuts or tears, both internally and externally, about the genitals or anus, or both
- bleeding from within the vagina, anus or penis, or the discharge of other body fluids that are foreign to the child
- discharge from vagina or anus of foreign fluids or articles
- skin damage around the mouth
- contracting a sexually transmitted disease (STD)
- urinary disease or infection
- becoming pregnant.

Discomfort

Sexual abuse may not result in a physical injury but may cause continual discomfort and pain. Symptoms may be:

- abdominal pain – with no obvious specific cause or recognisable injury
- discomfort while running, walking or while seated

- persistent pain or discomfort in the genital and anal area
- pain whilst urinating or defacating.

Pregnancy

Pregnancy can obviously be as a result of rape but also may result from willing sexual intercourse participation by the adolescent female (although, in this circumstance, an offence of Indecent Assault by Penetration is committed – not rape). However, major concern must be raised when the adolescent female is pre-teenage or early teenage and in particular when the female concerned is very secretive about the father.

Contracting a sexually transmitted disease (STD)

It is obvious that a child having contracted a sexually transmitted disease is highly likely to have experienced some form of sexual abuse. The sexual activity is likely to include vaginal or anal sexual intercourse (penile penetration) or oral sexual activity.

Contracting a urinary tract infection (UTI)

Urinary tract infections are commonly caused by sexual activity. If diagnosed in a child, consideration should be given to sexually abusive behaviour.

Behavioural symptoms

Knowledge of sexual matters is too advanced for the age of the child

This may include the following.

- Child using words or phrases associated with sexual behaviour that would not normally be used by a child of his or her years (e.g. a five-year-old child using words or phrases like orgasm, penis, sex, making love, wank, etc.).
- Child describing sexual behaviour that he or she has witnessed or in which he or she has participated; again not expected at the child's age (e.g. 'white stuff coming out the end of his willy', 'Daddy lying on top of mummy and moving up and down' or 'saw picture of men and women with no clothes on, he and I then did the same').
- Sexual awareness can also be expressed through a child's drawing or through displays of sexual simulation when playing with dolls.

Sexualised behaviour displayed by a young child

This may include:

- children kissing adults or other children on the lips in a sexually passionate fashion as opposed to a platonic, friendly fashion; may also include the knowledge and ability to 'French kiss'

- a five-year-old boy rubbing his hands over the chest of a five-year-old girl
- a four-year-old boy rubbing his own genitalia as if masturbating
- a child of any age acting as if educating other children in sexual matters
- a seven-year-old boy pulling a seven-year-old girl to the ground, lying on top of her and moving in such a fashion as to unwittingly simulate sexual intercourse
- an eight-year-old boy pulling down the knickers of a six-year-old girl and rubbing her genitalia
- a female child, during normal play with other children, lying down on her back and spreading her legs, emulating the missionary position, as if to encourage or engage in sexual intercourse.

Over-sexualised behaviour towards adults

A younger child, not being socially aware of the implications or acceptability of his behaviour, may act towards all or a selected number of adults in an overly sexualised fashion. The behaviours may include:

- touching adults about the genital area or about the breasts
- the child inserting his tongue into the mouth of an adult or other child when kissing, or making passionate mouth or body movements when kissing
- the child lifting certain clothing worn by adults or other children
- the child unfastening his or others' clothing to, or to simulate, the exposure of genitals or breasts
- striking seductive poses.

The performing of these sexualised behaviours is of far greater concern if the child in question attempts or is successful in accomplishing them in a covert or guarded fashion.

Running away

A child may feel that the only way to avoid abuse, or to have it stop, will be to run away from the environment in which the abuse occurs. The child may run away for a short time or hide near to home in the hope that the attention drawn will stop the abuse. Conversely, the child may run away and never return, fearful of the reprisal from her abuser.

It is most likely that the child will run away to local friends and be found. This behaviour may be repeated several times before the abuse is finally identified.

Isolates oneself from peers

A child suffering sexual abuse may be fearful that other children will identify the abuse and harmfully cause ridicule. The child may also feel that other children will want to talk about the experience in a friendly manner, but this reminds the child of the pain and hurt and therefore distances him- or herself from other children to avoid the possibility.

The sexually abused child is also unlikely to be keen or interested in interacting normally with other children because of the constant preoccupation with the abuse. The playing of games, singing of songs and the completion of schoolwork are likely activities in which a sexually abused child will not wish to become engaged. If the child is forced to engage, it is likely that he or she will fail to excel due to poor concentration.

Fear of being naked among peers

Often, a child experiencing sexual abuse becomes self-conscious about his or her own body and will fear being seen naked. This is due in many cases to the child feeling different from all the other children and fearful that what is actually an imaginable physical sign will be noticed and that he or she will be ridiculed. As a result, many sexually abused children will go to great lengths to avoid being in situations where they can be seen naked in front of others, such as school or public communal changing areas.

Has a fear of certain adults

One family member or one family friend may be the current abuser of the child. In this case, the child may well act normally around other adults within the family group, but behave quite differently when the abuser is present. The child may not speak out about the abuse, but shy away, doing all that is possible in order to distance him- or herself from the abuser. In addition, the child may display an unusual behaviour when in the presence of the abuser, although parents or carers may not understand this behaviour and believe that the child is merely shy, being naughty or simply seeking attention.

Displays hostility

A sexually abused child may display high levels of anger, hatred or aggression towards adults and other children whether or not the adults or children are known to the child. This behaviour may erupt without there being any obvious catalyst such as bullying, taunting, imposing discipline, etc. The hostility displayed by the child is very likely to remain constant while the abuse continues, with the child being unlikely to explain to a carer why he or she is acting in this fashion during that period.

Becomes badly behaved and achievements at nursery/school deteriorate

The child may simply become ill behaved, disruptive and disobedient. As a result, nursery or schoolwork will deteriorate. This may include written work, spelling, sporting activities, arts and crafts, etc. This may be out of character and indicate an initial stage of abuse.

Kills or harms the family pet

Research has shown that sexually abused children may well vent their fear, anger or frustration on another living creature. As the victim is unlikely to kill or harm another member of the family, particularly the abuser, the victim will possibly attack the family's or neighbour's defenceless pet.

Sleep patterns are disturbed

A sexually abused child may display symptoms of extreme tiredness or even exhaustion, resulting from the experience of restless or sleepless nights either in fear of further abuse, or from suffering stress relating to the current abuse. Exhaustion may cause the child to fall asleep at unusual or unnatural times and develop irregular sleeping patterns.

Eating habits deteriorate and eating patterns are disturbed

The child may disregard his or her educated eating habits and begin to eat with little in the way of manners. Types of food that the child likes may change and the quality of preferred food may deteriorate so the child begins eating little else but junk food such as crisps and sweets. The eating timetable may also change with the child eating at bizarre or irregular times of the day.

Telling lies

A child who becomes the victim of sexual abuse, who has acquired a perfect history for honesty, may suddenly change and begin to tell stupid lies, which are easily identifiable. The child's skill in lying may well develop and as time passes the child may enter a complete fantasy world. Ultimately, the child may lie to such an extent, and with such plausibility, that the child begins to believe its fantasy world is real. The child is unlikely to disclose the real reason why he or she is lying and may possibly give a false explanation.

Fake illnesses or true but unexplained illnesses (psychosomatic)

A child suffering sexual abuse will often fake an illness for a variety of reasons. These may include:

- to avoid being at a place where the abuser will have access to the child, e.g. school, youth club, family gathering, place of part-time work, etc.
- to avoid being out in the community as the child may have a fear of falling prey to another abuser
- to purposefully draw attention to oneself in the hope that abuse will be identified, should the child not have the courage to speak out
- to avoid having to face peers or people in authority as the child wishes to be introvert and become isolated.

A child may also display signs of an illness that cannot be explained. This is known as a psychosomatic illness. It is an illness brought about by the child's mental or emotional state rather than by any physical factors.

Persistent masturbation

An older child who is being sexually abused, but has also experienced pleasurable sexual activity (e.g. a 14-year-old male having sexual intercourse with a willing 15-year-old female – an unlawful act due to age), may wish to continue experiencing sexual pleasure. As the child is uncertain or unclear emotionally as to what he or she should do, or wishes not to engage in sexual activity with the abuser, he or she may well begin to masturbate with alarming regularity.

Also, an abuser may well encourage or instruct a younger child to masturbate frequently. This will be in an effort to reduce the child's embarrassment or self-consciousness when later engaging in any form of sexual activity with the abuser.

Anxiety, depression

Sexual abuse, like any other form of abuse, can induce anxiety and clinical depression. If a child is diagnosed by a medical practitioner as suffering anxiety or clinical depression, the possibility that the child is being subjected to continued sexual abuse should not be dismissed.

Initial disclosure of the abuse is likely to be partial and not wholly convincing

For a child, disclosing sexual abuse to a family member, a friend or teacher, will probably be the greatest challenge the child will have ever had to undertake. The child will probably be very concerned about the outcome of the disclosure, particularly if the abuser has made violent threats towards the child or towards the child's parents, if he or she should disclose the abuse to the authorities. The child is also likely to fear not being believed, thinking they will be either admonished or ridiculed.

References

Angus G, Woodward S. *Child Abuse and Neglect Australia 1993–94*. Child Welfare Series No. 13. Canberra: Australian Institute of Health and Welfare, AGPS. Quoted in: National Child Protection Clearinghouse. *Update on Child Sexual Abuse*. Issues in Child Abuse Prevention, Number 5, Summer 1995. www.aifs.gov.au/nch/issues5.html

Department of Health. *Working Together to Safeguard Children – a guide to inter-agency working to safeguard and promote the welfare of children*. London: Department of Health; 2006. http://www.everychildmatters.gov.uk/resources-and-practice/IG00060

Kempe RS, Kempe CH. *Child Abuse*. London: Fontana/Open Books; 1978. Quoted in: National Child Protection Clearinghouse. *Update on Child Sexual Abuse*. Issues in Child Abuse Prevention, Number 5, Summer 1995. www.aifs.gov.au/nch/issues5.html

Schechter MD, Roberge L. Sexual exploitation. In: Helfer RE, Kempe CH (eds) *Child Abuse and Neglect: the family and the community*. Cambridge: Ballinger; 1976.

9

Recognisable signs of a child suffering neglect

What is child neglect?

By definition it is:

Neglect *adj* to treat with no regard, inattentive or negligent to do what should be done.

In 1999 the Department of Health produced a guide entitled *Working Together to Safeguard Children – a guide to inter-agency working to safeguard and promote the welfare of children*; the guide was revised in 2006. All the following relevant references are taken from the revised edition.

In the Department's guide, the term neglect is described as follows:

Neglect is the persistent failure to meet a child's basic physical and/or psychological needs, likely to result in the serious impairment of the child's health and development. Neglect may occur during pregnancy as a result of maternal substance abuse. Once a child is born, neglect may involve a parent or carer failing to provide adequate food and clothing, shelter including exclusion from the home or abandonment, failing to protect a child from physical and emotional harm or danger, failure to ensure adequate supervision including the use of inadequate care-takers, or the failure to ensure access to appropriate medical care or treatment. It may also include neglect of, or unresponsiveness to, a child's basic emotional needs. (Department of Health 2006)

The neglect of a child may also occur when an adult or other carer is guilty of one or more of the following:

- failing to wash or bath the child
- providing unclean clothing and an unhealthy, unclean living environment
- failing to teach the child necessary yet basic skills for adult life (speech, toilet-training, dressing, etc.)
- allowing the child to enter or remain in a dangerous situation with or without supervision (playing near a busy roadway, unsupervised bathing, exposing child to inappropriate and/or incompetent supervision/babysitters)
- knowingly allowing the child to be cared for by an adult or other child that poses a physical, emotional or sexual threat to the child.

The Home Office's *Working Together to Safeguard Children* continues, outlining the possible impact of neglect:

> Severe neglect of young children has adverse effects on children's ability to form attachments and is associated with major impairment of growth and intellectual development. Persistent neglect can lead to serious impairment of health and development, and long-term difficulties with social functioning, relationships and educational progress. Neglected children may also experience low self esteem, feelings of being unloved and isolated. Neglect can also result, in extreme cases, in death. The impact of neglect varies depending on how long children have been neglected, the children's ages, and the multiplicity of neglectful behaviours children have been experiencing. (Department of Health 2006)

Note
Neglected children are by far the most likely to become victims of sexual abuse by adults. They crave attention, love, physical contact (cuddles), gifts of clothing, toys and games, etc. They are easily identifiable by the predatory paedophile and regularly targeted. Emotionally and physically neglected children can be easily persuaded to accept gifts and acts of supposed kindness; the result being that the child 'prefers' the company of the paedophile over its own parents or carers.

Child neglect is sometimes very difficult to identify when working with children from various social backgrounds. Often, a child may look uncared for by virtue of poor clothing or unkempt appearance; however, the child may be from a low-income family where the parents are not able to provide their children with the clothes they desire. The child may also be from a background where personal appearance is not a major issue.

A neglected child may display any one of the following

In most cases of child neglect, more than one of the following characteristics is present.

Being underweight for height or small for age (stunted growth)

Parents, teachers and childminders all have an idea about the average size and weight of a healthy child relevant to their age. Significant underweight or short stature in a child may indicate neglect, although it is possible that illness is the cause.

Some children will suffer neglect later in life and will have grown correctly until the time that the neglect began. Such children may suddenly show signs of weight loss and/or the beginning of physical underdevelopment.

Having a pale complexion

A child suffering neglect may lose colour pigmentation in their skin and appear pale. This may be due to a number of reasons – lack of nourishment, worry, stress, upset or depression.

Poor hygiene

The child's skin and hair may be unwashed, resulting in skin disorders and a poor complexion, and they may have an unkempt appearance. They may suffer from untreated tooth decay and show little or no knowledge of personal body or oral hygiene.

If the child is very young, they may well constantly suffer from nappy rash. Clothes will be dirty, unwashed and odorous. The child may only be allowed a few clothes, and they may well be worn and need replacing.

Lacking lustre, listless, tired with little or no energy

Most happy, healthy children are full of life and 'bubbly' in character. A child suffering neglect will not display such zest. They will act and look 'dull' and will constantly appear tired and listless. They will have little or no interest in most things and will be very difficult to motivate, stimulate or to encourage.

Hunger

A neglected child may well show signs of hunger by overeating or displaying gluttony when offered food or drink. They may also hoard or steal food which belongs to other children. A hungry child is also very unlikely to share food or sweets with others.

Constantly suffering from minor illnesses

If a child is undernourished, maltreated, emotionally disturbed as a result of neglect, and/or generally performing below par, they are likely to contract minor illnesses such as colds, coughs, influenza or diarrhoea with alarming regularity.

Evidence of untreated illnesses and injuries

A neglected child may be sent to school, playgroup or childminder even when they are seriously ill or have a severe injury. It may become apparent, when talking with the child, that the parent or carer has not taken appropriate steps to obtain the necessary medical treatment for the child and the illness or injury has gone untreated. The result may be long-lasting illnesses or untreatable injuries.

Child often being kept at home and not attending school

There could be a number of reasons for a child regularly not attending school. The reasons could include:

- the parent or carer is uninterested in the child's educational welfare and therefore has little or no inclination or intention to take the child to school
- the parent or carer is maliciously withholding the child's opportunity to learn
- the parent or carer is concerned that the poor physical state of the child, giving obvious evidence of neglect, may well be identified by school staff or other parents.

Failure to interact with teachers and other adults

If a child appears happy when in the company of other children, but is frightened and timid when in the company of adults, they may well be suffering neglect and regular admonishment by their parent or carer if they complain. The child, in this instance, may be reluctant to interact with teachers, childminders or other adults.

In addition, a neglected child may have experienced emotional warmth, fondness or friendliness suddenly being taken away. By not interacting with their teacher or childminder, who may display such pleasantries, the child is shielding itself from the anguish and pain of losing such a bond and suffering the feelings of rejection.

The child may also feel that interacting with adults is worthless as they may view all adults in a similar light, and believe that teachers or childminders will display the same neglectful and callous attitude as the child's neglectful parents or carers.

Remaining at school after hours

A child suffering neglect may not wish to return home until it is absolutely necessary. They may loiter about the school premises long after school hours, though not engaging in any activity. The school is a familiar place that may provide warmth and safety to the child and they may have friends there, with whom to spend time.

Latching on to one adult – attention seeking

It is possible that one particular teacher or adult may 'connect' with the child and the child sees in that person what is lacking in their parents or carers. The child may constantly follow the chosen teacher or adult and continually seek attention from this one individual. The 'connecting' adult could be another family member, family friend or neighbour. As detailed in the Note above, the 'connecting' adult could be a potential abuser.

A noticeable change in both the child's appearance and responses, following a change of carers

If it is known that a child has recently undergone a change of carer (e.g. new foster parents) and that since the change the child's physical appearance, state of alertness, attitude, behaviour, concentration level, ability to interact with others, etc., has suddenly improved, it is possible that the previous carers were neglecting the child.

Reference

Department of Health. *Working Together to Safeguard Children – a guide to inter-agency working to safeguard and promote the welfare of children*. London: Department of Health; 2006. http://www.everychildmatters.gov.uk/resources-and-practice/IG00060

Section Two conclusion

It must be remembered that a child may experience a non-abuse event, an emotion, a psychological or physical development, a dream, any conscious fantasy or suffer an illness or disability, or any combination of these events, which can lead to the presentation of the majority of the symptoms outlined in this section. A solitary symptom does not always prove abuse. In most cases, a series or combination of symptoms will indicate the likelihood of an abuse type, but careful analysis of the child's overall circumstance, behavioural pattern and an assessment of any injuries must be conducted before any judgement is made.

Child protection (children in need)

The 2006 Department of Health's publication *Working Together to Safeguard Children* reads:

> Children who are defined as being 'in need' under Section 17 of the Children Act 1989, are those whose vulnerability is such that they are unlikely to reach or maintain a satisfactory level of health or development, or their health and development will be significantly impaired, without the provision of services (section 17(10) of the Children Act 1989), plus those who are disabled. The critical factors to be taken into account in deciding whether a child is in need under the Children Act 1989 are what will happen to a child's health or development without services being provided, and the likely effect the services will have on the child's standard of health and development. Local Authorities have a duty to safeguard and promote the welfare of children in need. (Department of Health 2006)

Child protection (significant harm)

The 2006 Department of Health's publication *Working Together to Safeguard Children* reads:

> Some children are in need because they are suffering or likely to suffer significant harm. The Children Act 1989 introduced the concept of significant harm as the threshold that justifies compulsory intervention in family life in the best interest of children, and gives local authorities a duty to make enquiries to decide whether they should take action to safeguard or promote the welfare of a child who is suffering, or likely to suffer significant harm.
>
> A court may make a care order (committing the child to the care of the local authority) or supervision order (putting the child under the supervision of a social worker, or a probation officer) in respect of a child if it is satisfied that:

- the child is suffering, or is likely to suffer, significant harm; and
- that the harm or likelihood of harm is attributable to a lack of adequate parental care or control (s.31).

There are no absolute criteria on which to rely when judging what constitutes significant harm. Consideration of the severity of ill-treatment may include the degree and the extent of physical harm, the duration and frequency of abuse and neglect, the extent of premeditation, and the presence or degree of threat, coercion, sadism, and bizarre or unusual elements. Each of these elements has been associated with more severe effects on the child, and/or relatively greater difficulty in helping the child overcome the adverse impact of the maltreatment. Sometimes, a single traumatic event may constitute significant harm, e.g. a violent assault, suffocation or poisoning. More often, significant harm is a compilation of significant events, both acute and long standing, which interrupt, change or damage the child's physical and psychological development. Some children live in family and social circumstances where their health and development are neglected. For them, it is the corrosiveness of long-term emotional, physical and sexual abuse that causes impairment to the extent of constituting significant harm. In each case, it is necessary to consider any maltreatment alongside the family strengths and supports. (Department of Health 2006)

To understand and establish significant harm, it is necessary to consider:

- the family context
- the child's development within the context of their family and wider social and cultural environment
- any special needs, such as medical condition, communication difficulty or disability that may affect the child's development and care within the family
- the nature of harm, in terms of ill-treatment or failure to provide adequate care
- the impact on the child's health and development *and*
- the adequacy of adult care.

It is important always to take account of the child's reactions, and his or her perceptions, according to the child's age and understanding.

Issues for parents to consider

Four main types of child abuse exist – emotional abuse, physical abuse, sexual abuse, and neglect. Either one or more can be exerted upon a child by either an adult or another child. On occasions, one abuse type may overlap another, not necessarily because a child understandably experiences an emotional disturbance while suffering physical abuse, but by the perpetrator inflicting upon the child specific suffering of a physical and emotional nature which ultimately causes physical harm and emotional upset.

Many ailments, injuries, behaviours and conditions are indicative of either of these abuse types, but not all are obvious or clearly noticeable; on occasions, the symptoms of emotional and sexual abuse are the most difficult to recognise.

Normal day-to-day observations of a child in a routine family environment, or within a care-home situation, should allow for a parent or carer to recognise some if not all of the symptoms of abuse displayed by the child, should he or she become a victim.

A child suffering any form of abuse will display one symptom or more which can be identified by family members or carers who are in daily contact with the child. The symptoms can vary between abuse types, and apart from obvious signs of physical injury, disease or pregnancy, will be in one of the following forms:

- a change in attitude
- an alteration in appearance
- changes in the way in which the child responds to change
- changes in the way in which the child reacts to disappointment
- changes in the way in which the child accepts discipline
- a change in the way the child approaches or responds to certain adults.

Reference

Department of Health. *Working Together to Safeguard Children – a guide to inter-agency working to safeguard and promote the welfare of children*. London: Department of Health; 2006. http://www.everychildmatters.gov.uk/resources-and-practice/IG00060

Section Three

The Internet – dangers and safeguards

10

Children using the Internet – information parents should know

The Internet is a fantastic tool

The Internet is a virtual world in which information relating to any subject can be easily, and usually freely, found. The latest pictures from the Hubble space-telescope, images from the depths of our deepest oceans, worldwide botany, pornography, ancient and recent history, anatomy, business and commerce, racing-car developments, past and present wars, politics, games, school and university educational programmes, holidays, law, financial advice and bank-ing – these are a few examples of the many thousands of subjects that are available to the Internet user; for viewing, and very often online interaction. In addition, thousands of retail companies and traders offer their goods for sale through online shopping, with many offering discounted prices and prod-uct reviews.

The Internet is, by its very nature, an absorbing phenomenon. It is easy for anyone to sit in front of a computer screen and pass several hours simply scanning the variety of topics on which information is available, let alone focus upon one topic and research that topic fully. It is also very easy to explore and search the Internet in great depth. As knowledge of Internet workings increases, the user will develop skills enabling enhanced use of search engines and search parameters; and, with greater precision, be able to locate a far greater amount of chosen information.

All the subjects detailed above and more are available to anyone who can gain access to the Internet – great if you, the user, know how to use the Internet and are looking to research the life and times of Queen Elizabeth I, or the demise of the Inca Civilisation. However, if you have little knowledge or experience in the workings of the Internet and Internet navigation, problems can soon arise. If you begin searching wildly for information relating to your chosen subject, it is quite possible that at some stage you will encounter an 'offer' to view adult pornography or an adult-themed site. On rare occasions, you may even experi-ence accidental exposure to adult pornography as no offer or warning is given and immediate access to sexually explicit images is forced upon you. As an example, I once searched for information on Queen Elizabeth I. I simply entered 'Queen Elizabeth I' in the search box of my chosen search engine and was presented with numerous websites which included one called 'images of the first Elizabeth'. I accessed this site and was confronted with a video clip of an adult female dressed as Queen Elizabeth I dancing a striptease (the site is no longer active). In this instance, the images contained within the clip would be described as 'soft porn' and did not cause any distress. However, more worrying imagery has been known to appear without warning.

What is more worrying for parents is the very real prospect that, while seeking to 'chat' with another genuine user, you or your child may unwittingly converse with a targeting, predatory paedophile.

Many children and teenagers make great use of the Internet as it offers fantastic entertainment and an opportunity to communicate with friends and family both near and far. It is also offers wonderful study programmes and can be utilised as an education tool at all levels. Its ability to quickly and clearly provide access to information on any subject to assist with homework, coursework and projects is unquestionable, and the depth of its resource is virtually unbound. Most schools in the UK use computers, and have information technology (IT) and Internet use as part of their curriculum with pupils and students tasked to use the Internet for both IT skill development and researching source material. It is worth remembering that both school pupils and college students are therefore more likely to be aware of the most up-to-date computer technologies and Internet advances – invariably, surpassing the computer and Internet knowledge of their parents or carers. To most children, worldwide communication is fascinating, and the prospect of being able to send photographs, live video or information to another person halfway around the world instantaneously and build a catalogue of international contacts, can be addictive.

The user's development of Internet skills and knowledge is also true of communication and 'chat'. One begins with simple e-mailing – a message sent from one computer to another. 'Chat' is totally different. Chat rooms are cyber-locations within the Internet where users can link with one or more other users and communicate in 'real time'. In other words, as one user types a word or sentence, the recipient can read what is written immediately and can respond instantaneously, almost as if verbally communicating. But that's not all; individual users can send 'text' to a chat room using a mobile phone and, with the use of headsets and web-cams, users can actually see and talk to each other via the Internet. One established and reputable search engine has developed a completely free system, whereby verbal communication can be made anytime, anywhere in the world, between users.

Some chat rooms are dedicated to particular subjects while others are open for all to use and converse on any given subject. They exist in a number of formats and are available on various computer networks. They can be found as:

- Internet Relay Chat (IRC). This is not too dissimilar to Citizen Band (CB) radio. This is the most popular of all chat-room services and is not owned or managed by any one organisation.
- Interactive 'role-play' environments. These are chat rooms that form part of online games.
- Web-based chat. Most Internet Service Providers (ISPs) such as AOL, BT or Freeserve, or Internet Portals such as Yahoo! or MSN, offer chat-room facilities.
- Independent or private chat rooms. Any individual user or group that possesses a website can offer the services of a chat room.
- Mobile phone use. Increasingly, mobile phone users are able to access chat rooms and communicate freely.

If two Internet users have a pre-arranged agreement to go 'online' at a given time and enter a specific chat room, or know each other's chat-room 'name', they are likely to communicate with one another in a 'safe environment'. Difficulties and concerns can arise when a genuine user enters a chat room and begins communicating and developing a 'cyber-relationship' with a person who is unknown to them.

It is a concerning and sobering thought that your child can so easily encounter a skilled, predatory, grooming and determined paedophile, without even leaving the house. You may ask, 'what harm can be done if my child's contact is solely through the computer?' The answer is simply this: most paedophiles will stop at nothing to gain physical access to children and will seductively entice your child into acting in a fashion you would never have conceived possible – even ignoring common sense, ignoring rules set between you, and willingly or unwillingly meeting the 'abusing user' in private.

Safety for adolescent and child users of the Internet

Underestimating a child's Internet usage and exposure to pornography

UK Children Go Online: in July 2004, the Economic and Social Research Council funded an investigation into Internet usage with co-funding from AOL, BSC, Childnet-International, Citizens Online and ITC. Its aim was to establish the typical use of the Internet and its impact upon 9- to 19-year-olds. In order to achieve this, the Council conducted a national, in-home, face-to-face survey lasting some 40 minutes, of 1,511 9- to 19-year-olds and 906 parents of the 9- to 19-year-olds. The following statistics, produced in 'UK Children Go Online'(April 2005), are just a few of the many concerning statistics relating to Internet usage by young people:

- 75% have Internet access in the home
- 19% have Internet access in their own bedroom
- 92% have Internet at school
- 41% utilise the Internet daily
- 43% utilise the Internet weekly
- 38% trust most of the information on the Internet
- 57% of the 9- to 19-year-olds who go online once a week have come into contact with online pornography
- 38% have seen a pornographic pop-up advertisement while conducting other Internet activities
- 36% have accidentally found themselves on a pornographic website while conducting other Internet activities
- 25% have received pornographic junk mail or e-mail or by instant messaging
- parents underestimate children's negative experiences: 33% of daily and weekly users have received unwanted sexual or nasty comments online or by text message, though only 7% of parents are aware that their child has received sexual comments (UK Children Go Online April 2005 – ESRC July 2004).

The basics that parents need to learn

Parents and carers of children utilising the Internet should make every effort, for both their and their children's benefit, to become conversant with the workings of the Internet and knowledgeable in the following areas:

- rudimentary understanding of the Internet and its usage within the home, at school and at Internet cafés
- what is available on the Internet – what is immoral, illegal or unethical
- what are:
  - Instant Messenger Programs
  - parental controls
  - blocks and filters
  - chat rooms both moderated and non-moderated (moderated chat rooms are chat rooms which are monitored by staff employed by the ISP who oversee the communication and content of text and images communicated between users).

All the up-to-date information concerning these topics is available from your Internet Service Provider (ISP). Various websites are accessible that detail advice, recommend safety issues and offer software to help educate the novice user (*see* Appendix B). In addition, many books are available that explain the complete workings of the Internet.

Parents and carers really should consider investing time and money in learning how the Internet works. Also, they should consider speaking with staff at schools and colleges to ascertain what security levels are imposed in their organisation, concerning Internet access and child users.

Safeguards and rules for children

The following is directed to children and adolescents, but is also essential reading for parents and guardians.

All family members utilising the Internet should be taught and encouraged to maintain the following.

Start up

- If, as a family unit, you are new to the Internet or changing your Internet Service Provider (ISP), it is advantageous for an adult to be present when a child creates his or her 'Chat Room Personal Profile'. When the ISP requests personal details, consider carefully the type of information you and your child supply. What may appear to you as 'innocuous details' may be sufficient for a targeting paedophile to identify your child's true name, address, school or other family members. Most ISPs will have information upon how best to create a safe profile. The following are a few suggested personal details listed as either safe or unsafe to circulate when engaging in Internet chat.

Safe:
– personally chosen Internet chat-room name (not personal name or e-mail name)
– home address region, e.g. South West, Midlands or North East
– brief description of interests, e.g. football, reading, art or camping.

Unsafe:
– true own name and names of family members
– own nickname that is established among peer group
– unusual or unique names of family members, friends or pets
– house number or house name, road name, village or city district or town of own address
– school name
– school address
– club or association name and address
– personal physical description
– photograph, depicting oneself, family members or local locations
– holiday destinations and locations of past holidays if visited regularly.

- Keep passwords secure. Do not divulge to friends or family members.
- Agree to have parents or carers informed of the names and other known personal details of all contacts with whom the child-user converses – NO SECRETS. This can be achieved by the user informing his or her parents or carers of the new contact's user name, nickname, chat-room name, interests, unusual vocabulary or terminology, addresses or locations and photograph. Obviously, a great deal will depend upon the volume and nature of the information supplied by the user, but consideration should be given to all aspects of communicated information.
- Agree to have parent or carers notified when a child-user is about to enter a chat room.
- Agree to leave a chat room immediately the child-user is sent or identifies any material that is suggestive, threatening or generally makes the child-user feel concerned or uncomfortable.
- Agree that parent or carers have complete access to any material stored on the family computer's hard drive or other data-saving media – AGAIN, NO SECRETS.

Continued use

- Users should never divulge any personal information in response to unsolicited e-mail, web pages, pop-ups, linked advertisements or, most importantly, non-personally known online contacts. The type of information usually sought by targeting paedophiles is described below.
NEVER DIVULGE ANY OF THE FOLLOWING INFORMATION:
 – true name
 – date of birth
 – details of home address, not even the name of the town where you live
 – contact telephone numbers (landlines or mobiles)
 – schools attended, be that details of either current school, past schools or college likely to be attending in the future
 – names and locations of any clubs attended or membership of any association

- location/s where child plays, associates with other children, etc., or any other location where the child-user could be vulnerable to approach by the paedophile.
- Never send credit card or banking details to an online contact.
- Never forward a personal photographic image or personal detailed description to an online contact, unless the recipient is personally known and parents or carers give consent.
- Always check the e-mail header for unusual wording or layout.
- Do not open e-mails or attachments unless you are aware of the sender and trust them. Such e-mails or attachments could contain viruses or other software that may assist the sender in identifying a child's identity and location.
- If the child-user receives messages that are sexually explicit or sexually suggestive, agree that parents should be informed immediately. If indecent images are received, parents or carers should report the matter to their Internet Service Provider and the police.
- Check unsolicited e-mails or web pages for spelling or grammatical errors.
- If you intend to visit public areas of the Internet and engage in communication, create an e-mail address that is different from that used by family members for communicating with friends and other family.
- Never respond to SPAM (Internet junk mail) as replying confirms your e-mail address to the sender.
- Utilise a SPAM filter to block unsolicited e-mails.
- Never download or open an attachment to an e-mail unless you are fully aware of the sender.
- Utilise pop-up blocking software that most Internet Service Providers offer freely for use.
- Employ the available and appropriate parental controls.
- Allow your children to access only 'moderated' chat rooms.

Gifts

- Do not accept gifts, of any kind, from individuals who are personally unknown and are solely online contacts, irrespective of the period over which the Internet relationship has been established. These include gifts posted to you (though you should never divulge your home address) and gifts e-mailed or sent as data packages, e.g. music, software or information. Paedophiles who attempt to groom children via the Internet can gain power and control by presenting a child-user with numerous gifts, on the initial understanding that they are free. Suddenly the paedophile changes tack and demands that the child-user pay for the gifts. This may cause the child-user to feel indebted and to reveal information or act in an unfamiliar way, which would never be normally considered.
- In addition, the paedophile may begin to commit acts of blackmail and force a child-user to reluctantly act inappropriately.

Web-cams

- If a child-user intends to send a photograph or converse with a contact utilising a web-cam, consider who is actually the recipient; the contact may 'write' that she is 15 years of age (the same as the user perhaps) and also likes the latest pop group, but the contact could be a 55-year-old man, with a sexual liking for 13 to 15-year-old girls. He may reside 300 miles away; he may reside in a neighbouring street.

- If using a web-cam, consider what can be seen in the image you are presenting. For example:
  - The camera, traditionally sited on top of the computer monitor, could be at such an angle that certain parts of a child-user's body are exposed.
  - Consider what clothing will be worn by the user when online. Unfortunately, some paedophiles will meaningfully misinterpret images and read into situations or circumstances what they are hoping for. The wearing of a nightdress by a child-user as the child goes online for 10 minutes before bed could create in the mind of a targeting paedophile that the child is seeking to entice a contact into bed with them. (Parents and guardians – *see* Chapter 5.) As a further example, the wearing of a bikini top by a nine-year-old girl, even though it may be the height of summer, might not be wise if the child-user is unfortunate enough to be unwittingly conversing with a 37-year-old male who likes pre-pubescent girls.
  - Backdrop – located behind the child-user may be photographs, personal items or a view from a window that will assist the paedophiliac user in identifying the child's address or location, and increase his chances of physically locating the child. Be mindful of what is displayed; besides, a child may not want the whole world to see the contents of an untidy bedroom.

Important note

When your computer is switched on, but your web-cam is not, make certain it is facing a wall or is covered. Software programs are available which allow unscrupulous Internet users to electronically enter your computer and switch your camera on, leaving you vulnerable to being viewed without your knowledge.

A golden rule for children

Do not arrange to physically meet any person with whom you have established a friendship through an internet chat room, even if the friendship has been maintained for a considerable time and the contact has become a 'keypal'. Discuss this issue with your parent or carer.

Safeguards and actions for parents

Monitor the behaviour of your child or adolescent. Draw comparisons between access to online and non-online pornography, and sexually abusive images of children.

Most adolescent males and a lesser number of adolescent females will, at some point, view or attempt to view adult pornography; an even smaller number will view sexually abusive images of children. Adolescents who choose to view sexually abusive images of children will not automatically embark on a lifetime of child sexual abuse; their choice could be made simply on inquisitive grounds. However, the ease with which children can obtain access to abusive images of children is both shocking and concerning and increases the chances of an adolescent's psychosexual development and sexual understanding being immorally and perversely influenced.

In the past, most pubescent and post-pubescent adolescents wishing to view pornography did so by quickly glancing at 'forbidden' magazines in newspaper shops or even stealing the magazines for viewing at a later time. Such magazines invariably contained only 'soft-porn' and were, for most people, the only source of such material. Though completely inappropriate for adolescents, they did little to affect the psychosexual development and sexual understanding of well-adjusted, inquisitive adolescents. 'Hard-core' pornography was only available in 'adult shops' or on the black market, whereas sexually abusive images of children were only to be found on sale on the black market; though some 'adult shop' retailers would sell from 'under the counter'. Either way, they were sources unlikely to be accessed by children or adolescents.

The Internet has changed this situation completely. Adolescents of all ages with a little training and experience can master the complexities of Internet navigation and with ease locate both adult pornography and sexually abusive images of children. While many adolescents view adult 'soft-porn' pornography online, it is possible for those who choose to do so to view adult 'hard-core' pornography ranging from perverse heterosexual acts between adults to adult homosexual interaction, sadism, masochism and bestiality. For the determined, who are prepared to 'borrow' credit-card details, access can be gained to websites offering scenes of male and female rape, sexual humiliation, sexual torture and even murder with a sexual overtone. In addition, sufficient payment to the 'right' people can give access to websites offering both video and still images of child sexual and physical abuse.

Adolescents who are regularly exposed to such extreme sexually explicit material may well be traumatised as a result. This may induce a change in their view or outlook on sexual matters which in turn can possibly cause long lasting damage or re-structuring to their psychosexual development and sexual understandings. This may cause sexual frustration, confusion or a misconception of what is normally acceptable as sexual behaviour between consenting adults; such exposure may also have an adverse effect on future sexual preferences, sexual stimulation and relationships. For some, the exposure fuels their uncontrollable desire to learn and fantasise about the perverse sexual activity that adults can experience and develop. For others, from as young as the age of seven years, it may stimulate and assist in satisfying fantastical sexual needs concerning other children and adults, as well as encouraging action which may lead to committing sexual assault.

What are we concerned about?

> Prolonged exposure to pornography leads to a skewed perception of normal sexual activity . . . there should be concern for young people with a relatively narrow perspective who are exposed to frequent images such as sodomy, group sex, sadomasochistic practices, and bestiality. (Zillmann 2000)

Differences between magazines and the Internet

Major differences exist between these types of media and parents and carers should consider the changes that have occurred, perhaps since their own youth. The Internet offers far greater opportunities to view indecent, immoral and illegal material than magazines ever did and, in addition, creates a number of inherent problems. The following are some examples of the differences and problems that can arise.

- Ease of access to still and moving images depicting both adult 'soft-porn' pornography and extremely perverse adult sexual activity.
- Availability of still and moving images showing sexually abusive behaviour towards and involving children.
- The volume of material available.
- Accidental access to indecent images – many unwanted 'pop-ups' advertise pornography; and often, search parameters on any given search engine can reveal 'porn websites' or even open an indecent image. In addition, the opening of unwanted or unsolicited e-mails can unintentionally present the user with images depicting both adult and adolescent sexualised scenes.
- The viewing of certain types of perverse sexual behaviour including sexually abusive images of children can cause severe trauma.
- For a number of reasons and due to the ease of access, an adolescent may become addicted to viewing pornography.
- If addiction continues and is not treated, the incessant viewing of 'soft-porn' may make the subject boring and staid. This can lead addicted adolescents to view more outrageous material and venture into the world of perverse sexual practices; this could include viewing material showing sexually abusive images of children.
- By viewing a sexually abusive image of a child on a computer screen, you are 'making' an indecent image of a child and are thereby breaking the law. If such images are 'saved' onto a computer's hard disk or other computer data-saving media, you are 'possessing' indecent images of children and are, again, breaking the law. If you choose to send an indecent image of a child to another Internet user or post or fax or text an indecent photograph to another person, you are 'distributing' indecent images of children and are, again, breaking the law.

Monitoring your child's online activities

As outlined above, NO SECRETS.

Parents and guardians should have full access to any data saved by their child. This is not always easy to agree and not always easy to enforce as data can be concealed on hard-drives and CD-ROMs, floppy disks and memory sticks, the latter three being easily concealed. However, if data is accessible, the following should be considered and concerns should be raised, *if your child:*

- begins to collect very large amounts of 'soft-porn', either on the family computer or on other data-saving media (floppy disks, CD-ROMs, memory sticks, etc.) – particular concern should be raised if material is being secretly stored on data-saving media and hidden from others

- stores material on the family computer but utilises encryption software to preserve the secrecy of the material or contact
- is circulating pornographic images to friends or others in peer or other groups
- is continuously returning to the same site or sites and views pornographic images 'live-time' without downloading
- commences viewing and storing perverse, sexually explicit material
- possesses or views images from websites offering scenes depicting adults acting in a sexually violent or extremely degrading fashion towards each other, towards children or towards animals
- collects or views sexually abusive images of children

or

- is very secretive about Internet access and activities
- accesses the Internet against parents' or carer's wishes
- accesses the Internet away from home, e.g. Internet cafes or homes of friends
- becomes isolated from friends and peers, and becomes obsessed with Internet access
- wishes to have computer with Internet access in their own room, so as to be isolated from family members
- leaves the home address with a mobile telephone immediately after a session of Internet usage and talks on the mobile telephone for long periods in secret.

In addition, parents should:

- take note if their child, while using Internet chat rooms or mobile telephone, begins using a headset to converse with others. Internet 'groomers' often suggest this practice to minimise the likelihood of being overheard by others in the home or school or club
- regularly check that parental-control software is working correctly; in addition, make certain that it has not been purposefully disabled
- regularly check for new or unknown telephone numbers repeatedly appearing on the family home telephone bill.

Further concerns

Protecting your identity and privacy

For a number of reasons, primarily criminal, 'personal identity theft' is on the increase. Fraudsters have numerous ways of obtaining and utilising your personal details – one-way *phishing*. Phishers send hoax e-mails or encourage you to visit hoax pages on websites purporting to be from professional companies and will request validation of your existence by way of requesting details such as a clarifying e-mail, full name and address and bank details.

There are two main areas for great concern regarding child sex crime and identity cloning on the Internet:

- a potential offender may well wish to hide his identity and utilise the details of another person to gain credibility, plausibility, funding and anonymity
- an innocent person, whose identity has been cloned, may well find themselves being accused and possibly under investigation on suspicion of

accessing illegal indecent and abusive images of children, or attempting to contact and illegally 'groom' a child via the Internet.

For the psychological, moral, ethical and physical safety of children, the protection of identity and privacy is paramount.

References

UK Children Go Online. April 2005. (ESRC, July 2004.) www.children-go-online.net/

Zillmann D. *Sexual Offending on the Internet.* COPINE Project. University College Cork; 2000. www.innovationlaw.org/userfiles/page_attachments/Library/1/Quayle_1223740.ppt

11

Paedophiles using the Internet – targeting, grooming and entrapment

For the purposes of this chapter, the term 'abuser' will be used when refer-ring to people (male or female) who choose to use the Internet as a medium for contacting, manipulating and grooming children immorally and illegally.

The Internet is a very efficient tool – for contacting and grooming children

As outlined in Chapter 10, the Internet has a great deal to offer. The opportunity to learn and research any number of subjects, or to communicate worldwide with friends or family, to maintain and create business, or plan the next holiday; these are just a few of the thousands of working options available to the user.

Sadly, not everyone uses the Internet in a totally moral, ethical and legal fashion. Its misuse is widespread, and ranges from the dissemination of debilitating viruses to financial fraud, theft, sales scams and corruption. Internet-based criminal activity of greatest concern is the large-scale production, trading and distribution, downloading, possession and viewing of illegal 'child sexual abuse images' and 'child physical abuse images' (professionals often refer to such images as CSAIs – Child Sexual Abuse Images – and CPAIs – Child Physical Abuse Images), and online grooming, sometimes referred to as IIG – Internet Initiated Grooming.

Historically, obtaining such images was a costly and difficult practice. Sources were scant and risks of being caught were high. As the images concerned were mostly in the form of printed photographs, people producing, possessing and selling such images were vulnerable to exposure by undercover police officers and custom officials.

The Internet has changed this situation dramatically. No longer is the possession and the sale of such material an occupation for the few. Activity of this sort is now open to thousands of like-minded individuals who choose to hide behind a computer screen continuously scanning for stimulating and arousing illegal images, or who constantly seek to find potential future victims.

What the Internet can provide for the abuser

Exhaustive potential to contact prospective victims

In July 2005 the world's human population was just under 6.5 billion. Of this figure, over 938 million people, only 14.6%, were recorded as utilising the

Internet. In the European Union, however, at the same time, the population was recorded at over 460 million, with over 221 million utilising the Internet; that is a European Union user rate of 48%. Interestingly, the increase in Internet usage within the European Union from the year 2000 to 2005 is almost 140%.

These figures give rise to concern for any parent or child carer residing within the European Union (EU). They show that a far greater percentage of people residing in the European Union are using the Internet than in most other regions of the world; which means, statistically, a far greater chance of a parent or carer, or child, communicating online with a European-based paedophile. An additional concern is that as EU borders are becoming less obstructive, peripatetic paedophiles are being presented with an increasingly easy and less detectable opportunity to travel from one county to another, thereby reducing for themselves the likelihood of identification or apprehension when travelling to meet with an online contact.

These figures show that throughout the world a vast number of people including would-be child sex offenders have the opportunity to contact any number of children, or to contact any number of people who may lead to a contact with children. Contact may be in any of the following forms:

- with children; directly through chat rooms, school sites, children's clubs and sports clubs, websites or user groups of child-interest topics
- with parents; through chat rooms, dating agencies, school PTAs (parent–teacher associations) or governorships, educational organisations (adults completing childcare courses, etc.), websites or user groups of general interest, parent support groups and parents selling children's old toys or clothes
- with childminders; through advertisements for employment, training opportunities and networking groups.

Note
Demographic (population) numbers are based on data contained in the World Gazetteer website. Internet usage information comes from data published by Nielsen//Net Ratings, by the International Telecommunication Union and by other reliable sources.

Easy access to sexually abusive material

An Internet-connected computer can provide access to innumerable 'personal' or 'company' websites that offer child sexual abuse images. Access to the Internet is now widely available – from home computers, Internet cafés, the workplace, laptop computers with a 'wireless' network facility, and mobile phones.

Affordability

A home computer with Internet access can cost as little as a few hundred pounds, and with Internet Service Providers offering basic Internet access for less than 20 pounds a month, sitting at home continuously viewing thousands of child sexual abuse images is an inexpensive activity.

If one takes into consideration the outlay balanced against the return, even if the user has to pay for website access, the cost of viewing images is on average less than a penny for tens, or even hundreds, of images. Trading in indecent images is, of course, invariably free.

Volume and variety of material

One of the major advantages of using the Internet for the purposes of research or indeed any other form of activity is the volume and variety of material that is readily available. The same can be said of child sexual abuse images. Once established as an Internet user, and having accessed specific sites, an abuser can gain access to thousands of images, video clips and soundtracks, all depicting the sexual abuse of children.

It is not uncommon for one abuser to have stored either on his computer's hard drive, removable storage or on the Internet, over 40,000 separate child sexual abuse images. If a link or trade is arranged, any one user can gain access to all of these images.

Anonymity and protection

As an Internet user, an abuser is faceless. He can remain within his own 'cyber world' if he chooses not to engage in 'live-contacting'. He can converse with other users anywhere in the world and give them a completely false representation of himself. He can portray himself as a child, adolescent or adult, claim to be male or female and be of any age.

Software can be purchased and installed that protects the abuser from being traced by most other users. In the majority of cases, only the authorities can establish user identification by direct access to the abuser's ISP (Internet Service Provider) with various Acts of Parliament allowing lawful breaches of the Data Protection Act 1998.

What effect Internet usage, of a paedophiliac and/or hebephiliac nature, can have upon an abuser

Brings about changes in mood

Access to child sexual abuse images can stimulate sexual urges and create sexual arousal. It can motivate abusers to act, having increased their desire to sexually engage with children. Such images may remind the abuser of his true sexual preference and, if combined with a current lack of preferred sexual activity, may cause misery or depression. Conversely, the stimulation and arousal (which may lead to orgasm after masturbation) can create a mental state of euphoria and happiness.

Lowers inhibitions

An abuser may well be inhibited in his physical activity if he feels that his desires are unique or shared with a very small number of other people. He may well feel that he is alone and what he wants to accomplish is so outlandish, so socially unacceptable, that he couldn't possible carry out such activity without the highest risk of being caught. However, access to vast quantities of child sexual abuse images via the Internet may cause him to form the belief that he is not alone in having such desires, and that what he wishes to accomplish is not unique. In addition, he may feel that if many other men are acting as he wishes to, the possibility of him offending without detection is highly promising.

Once engaged in sexual offending against a child, an abuser viewing child sexual abuse images of an extreme nature may be inspired to carry out more severe abusive acts.

Increases fantasy world

In addition to explicit sexual fantasies experienced by many abusers, some abusers derive great pleasure from creating a complete fantasy world. This can involve creating a whole 'new' person in their mind's eye. This fictitious person will have a false name, age, description, address, school, interests, parents and family, method of speech (computer language) and cyber name. In essence, the fictitious person can be whoever the abuser wants to be, either in real life or in some delusional grandiose existence. To increase the intensity of the fantasy-world experience, the abuser may well develop and possess several fictitious characters, and present a different character for each contact or child victim that he is attempting to groom.

Enhances confidence

The Internet allows for easy networking and fast communication between abusers. This quick and fairly secure contact method can help build confidence and provide reassurance of an abuser's ability to conduct successful grooming and offending activity.

Validates and justifies (to the abuser) his needs and usage

The abuser can feel validated and justified in his feelings and beliefs of paedophilia or hebephilia if he sees others acting out what he wants to accomplish. It becomes acceptable, understandable, more realistic and reinforces the abuser's belief that he can achieve the same.

Grooming – what exactly do abusers do?

Children using the Internet innocently can make contact with anyone, and be contacted by anyone, while online. Abusers who choose to use the facilities of Internet chat rooms are not always who or what they purport to be. It is easy to tell lies online. Many paedophiles enter child-orientated chat rooms portraying themselves as a young person, giving a false name, age and gender, and on occasions sending or displaying photographs of the young person they are claiming to be. They learn the typical online chat terms and phrases, and make childlike or adolescent comments; all in an effort to disguise their true age and gender and to be accepted within the 'child chat-room sect'.

Short-term goals

Initially, paedophiles with the intention of making contact and establishing relationships with children via the Internet will access one or more of the thousands of Internet chat rooms which are specifically maintained for the interest of children. Once in a chat room, they will advertise and offer themselves as 'contacts' and therefore candidates for being an online friend or 'keypal'. In doing this, the abuser introduces his online name and contact details to any number of child Internet users who unwittingly stumble across him having ventured into a jointly used chat room.

It is interesting to note that the level of activity and effort made by the abuser to make and maintain contact with children will be proportionately dependent upon the outcome the abuser seeks to achieve from his online Internet usage. Some abusers have no other interest than to 'chat' with children while portraying themselves as a child or adolescent. The excitement of communicating with a child about child matters and interests is sufficient to fulfil the abuser's needs and fuel his fantasises. For others, the compelling and only thought in their mind is the ultimate goal of controlling a child to the point of forcing a meeting and subjecting the child to penetrative sexual abuse.

Having well-established 'contacts', and many of them, is the key to successful and continued online abusing, so the abuser will work hard to become a recognised, accepted and popular contact within a number of specific child-orientated chat rooms. Various skills and experience will assist the abuser in identifying vulnerable child-users as well as identifying vulnerable parents or carers. In addition, the online abuser will be constantly on the lookout for children who are seemingly willing to engage in sexualised online 'chat'.

Long-term goals

The paedophiliac abuser will have a number of long-term goals and aspirations which he will hope to achieve and maintain. These may vary from one abuser to the next, but will chiefly consist of the following:

- a consistent number of known child Internet users whom he can communicate with and maintain at various stages of the grooming process
- a constant supply of new contacts whom the abuser can assess as to the suitability for online grooming and possible future physical sexual abuse
- establish a relationship with a child that will one day escalate to either cyber sex, the supplying by the victim of online sexually explicit still or video images, or a meeting, which may result in physical sexual abuse
- develop skills to enhance his ability to attract and identify the most likely candidates for online and physical sexual abuse
- create a repeatable method of online activity by which the contacting, grooming, controlling and abusing of a child is not identified.

Subterfuge

Not all adult online abusers portray themselves as a child or an adolescent and claim to be of a different gender while communicating with children – but most do. As Internet Service Providers and other agencies become better equipped to combat online child abuse, adults entering a child-orientated chat room masquerading as a child will be less likely to succeed in communicating with a child for illicit purposes. This is largely due to the increasing number of 'protected' or 'moderated' sites. The majority of major ISPs offer 'protected' or 'moderated' chat rooms; these are chat rooms which are monitored by staff employed by the ISP who oversee the communication and content of text and images communicated between users.

Note

It is worth remembering, though, that a number of adult abusers have entered child-orientated chat rooms, have not disguised their real age and gender, and have successfully groomed and abused children.

A large number of online abusers have considered this issue and have made the decision to create a false image of themselves in the belief that, by appearing as a child or as an adolescent and perhaps appearing as a female rather than a male, they increase their chances of success. As a faceless contact, any number of falsehoods can be expressed in an attempt to gain the trust, respect and the online friendship of a child.

Online abusers have been known to create completely fictitious profiles for themselves in preparation for going online and communicating with children. These profiles have consisted of a host of bogus names, false ages, and dates of birth, names and ages of spurious siblings and parents, phoney details of schooling and school friends, fake addresses and 'home-town' locations and, to complete the job, a photograph of a child matching the false physical description.

Key points of typical online activity leading to the control of a child

- Creates a false identity for himself – consisting of false name, age, gender, background, schooling, friends and family.
- Gains access to the Internet and enters numerous child-orientated chat rooms and user groups.
- Creates a recognisable 'signature', by becoming known by many for his jokes, views, wayward approach to schooling or parents, and is generally an attractive contact for young people.
- Builds a database containing a complete dossier on each young person with whom he develops an online relationship.
- Establishes the likelihood of grooming success based upon the reactions and responses of child contacts – often by monitoring the reaction of the child contacts to receiving sexually explicit images or text.

- Develops an acceptable level of risk which he will not overstep and will continually assess the risk of exposure in every case, to a point of abandoning a particular target; again this will be based upon the reactions and responses of the child contacts.
- Identifies a suitable candidate for victimisation by online and/or contact sexual abuse.
- Gleans knowledge of his chosen victim's social group, either online or through school or local friends.
- Can impose himself upon the child victim at any time, either at the family home, via the child's school Internet access or arranged times at Internet cafés.
- Attempts to isolate the victim by undermining the victim's relationship with family and friends.
- Works towards being the child victim's only contact. This is often achieved by causing the child victim to experience acute paranoia by claiming the victim's friends and family are communicating with each other behind the victim's back, and that the victim has been ostracised from his or her peer chat group. In some instances, the abuser will obtain the victim's computer address book and communicate with the victim's friends and family, sending correspondence which causes unrest, disharmony, feuds or anger within the group.
- On occasions, abusers have been known to identify and select a child whom they find attractive and most suitable for 'offline' sexual abuse and, having established a method of secret postal communication, send the child victim a pre-paid mobile telephone. This allows the abuser to have isolated contact with the child victim, and a more secure method of communication. In addition, the abuser creates a situation whereby, once the phone has been accepted, the child victim is embroiled into the grooming process by 'willingly accepting a gift'. The 'gift' and the acceptance of the 'gift' can also be used at a later stage as part of a blackmail approach should the abuser wish to use blackmail as a form of control.
- Gains control of the child victim by seduction or fear. These methods can consist of plying the child victim with gifts; or the use of threats or blackmail.

What effect sexually abusive images have upon the abuser

Viewing, possessing and collecting sexually abusive images of children, and distribution

People – sex offenders or not – only look at and collect things in which they are interested or can make a profit. It is therefore reasonable to accept that a man, viewing and collecting a quantity of child sexual abuse images, has an interest in such activity; either in making a financial profit from the making and distribution of child sexual abuse images or, more likely, for sexual arousal, for fantasy fuelling or as an aid to masturbation.

Child sexual abuse images (still and moving) can:

- stimulate fantasy and fuel the masturbation thought process
- encourage and strengthen the urge to sexually offend
- create a positive attitude within the abuser by way of cognitively distorting the truth, that their fantasy is uncommon and socially unacceptable

- educate the abuser, insomuch as images can inform abusers of what restraints or equipment can be used, and what singular or multiple acts can be performed
- reinforce the belief in the abuser that the desire to commit sexual abuse of children is not a one-off experience that only happens to a few; but that, in fact, sexual abuse of children is a regular occurrence, is a worldwide practice, open to anyone and that the abuser is not alone in his deviant thoughts and desires.

Unbelievably, within paedophiliac circles, respect and admiration can be earned by both the volume and the severity of the content of child sexual abuse images that an abuser is willing to distribute. Some of the most 'respected' paedophiles distribute thousands of still images, video and audio clips, depicting some of the most disturbing, terrorising, perverse and debased behaviour towards children that one could possibly imagine.

It is not uncommon for an abuser to offer thousands of images and video or audio clips in exchange for other images, information or money. Information that is sought can vary, and abusers will trade images for one or more of the following:

- details of children thought to be suitable as future sexual abuse victims
- details of current sexual abuse victims who can be shared
- details of other abusers who have contact with a wealth of children thought to be suitable as future sexual abuse victims.

Organisations combating and disrupting the supply and demand for child sexual abuse images

The Paedophile Online Investigation Team

The National Crime Squad is considered the main lead in all tactical issues in the fight against child abuse on and via the Internet. In January 2003, to assist the National Crime Squad in this monstrous task, the Paedophile Online Investigation Team (POLIT) was created. POLIT, which performs a supporting and coordinating role, is a single point of contact within the UK for reactive and proactive national and international enquiries and investigations into Internet-related child abuse. Once informed of an investigation or enquiry, POLIT performs detailed research and the assessment and dissemination of any relevant intelligence to UK law enforcement organisations.

Internet Watch Foundation

The Internet Watch Foundation (IWF) was formed in 1996 as a result of the Internet Service Provider industry, the government and the police agreeing that a 'partnership approach' was best suited to combating the distribution of child sexual abuse images.

Specially trained staff working for the Foundation deal solely with illegal online content, which includes minimising the availability of:

- child abuse images hosted anywhere in the world
- criminally obscene content hosted within the UK
- incitement to racial hatred content hosted within the UK.

Members of the public and professionals alike can log on to the IWF web-site (*see* Appendix B, 'Useful contact details') and report, to the Foundation, website addresses which either offer or appear to offer illegal or immoral material, offer morally dubious connectivity between users or appear to entice young persons to engage in suspicious online communication.

The IWF is a charitable organisation which is funded by the EU and the UK Internet industry including Internet Service Providers, mobile telephone network operators and manufacturers, Content Service Providers, telecommunications and software companies and credit card bodies.

Child Exploitation and Online Protection

The Child Exploitation and Online Protection (CEOP) Centre was launched on 24 April 2006. Based in London, the CEOP unit, headed by the former Deputy Director General of the National Crime Squad Jim Gamble, brings together law enforcement officials, children's charity specialist workers and staff from various industries, in the fight against on- and off-line child abuse.

CEOP is a dedicated 24 hours a day, seven days a week resource for reporting online child sexual abuse. Staff at the centre focus their attention directly upon illegal Internet use, which can vary from online grooming, the sending of immoral or illegal e-mail content and immoral chat-room communication and activity (which may involve the use of computers and mobile telephones). In addition, CEOP staff work to trace online abusers and identify victims and potential victims.

The COPINE Project – Combating Paedophile Information Networks in Europe

The COPINE unit is housed in the Department of Applied Psychology, University College Cork, Ireland, and since 1997 has been actively researching the area of child sexual abuse on the Internet under the supervision of Professor Max Taylor. From the beginning, the sexual abuse project has taken a very broad approach to the problem, researching areas such as effective treatment for offenders, prevention, assessment of risk and trying to learn more about how and why abuse images are collected.

It was this latter strand that led to the setting up of a database of abuse images downloaded from the Internet in cooperation with local police agencies around the globe, as well as international organisations such as Interpol and the National Centre for Missing and Exploited Children (NCMEC). Under Professor Taylor's guidance, COPINE has become recognised as a world authority on abuse images distributed over the Internet.

One of the many aspects of the work conducted by the COPINE Project is the identification of child sex abuse victims and the locations where sexually abusive images or sound recordings are made (photographs, videos or sound recordings taken of sexual abuse scenes). Seized sexually abusive images are closely scrutinised and details of background scenes or images are noted and recorded. These items of information are cross-referenced and often many different victims are found to have been photographed or video-recorded at the same location. Similarly, soundtracks are compared for background noises (*see* COPINE website).

Grades of sexually explicit abusive images of children – based on COPINE typology

Since its origin, the COPINE Project has amassed thousands of images which are held within its reference database. The images depict children set in scenes of varying indecency, and in order to assist in the grouping of the severity of the indecency, the images are categorised from one to ten. When indecent images are seized from a suspect they are categorised using the COPINE typology and the categorisation is often used for the purposes of criminal investigation, prosecution and risk assessment. What is concerning is the fact the majority of the material seized can be accessed by the public.

The category system described in Table 11.1 extends and develops the Platform for Internet Content Selection (PICS) and the Recreational Software Advisory

Table 11.1 A typology of paedophile picture collections (source: Taylor *et al.* 2001).

Level	Name	Description of picture qualities
1	Indicative	Non-erotic and non-sexualised pictures showing children in their underwear, swimming costumes, etc., from either commercial sources or family albums; pictures of children playing in normal settings, in which the context or organisation of pictures by the collector indicates inappropriateness.
2	Nudist	Pictures of naked or semi-naked children in appropriate nudist settings, and from legitimate sources.
3	Erotica	Surreptitiously taken photographs of children in play areas or other safe environments showing either underwear or varying degrees or nakedness.
4	Posing	Deliberately posed pictures of children fully/partially clothed or naked (where the amount, context and organisation suggests sexual interest).
5	Erotic posing	Deliberately posed pictures of fully/partially clothed or naked children in sexualised or provocative poses.
6	Explicit erotic posing	Emphasising genital areas where the child is either naked, partially or fully clothed.
7	Explicit sexual activity	Involves touching, mutual and self masturbation, oral sex and intercourse by child, not involving an adult.
8	Assault	Pictures of children being subject to a sexual assault, involving digital touching, involving an adult.
9	Gross assault	Grossly obscene pictures of sexual assault, involving penetrative sex, masturbation or oral sex involving an adult.
10	Sadistic/bestiality	a Pictures showing a child being tied, bound, beaten, whipped or otherwise subjected to something that implies pain. b Pictures where an animal is involved in some form of sexual behaviour with a child.

Council (RSACi) rating system (Akdeniz, 1997), but more directly focuses on pictures related to adult sexual interest in children.

This categorising system quite deliberately includes pictures that do not fall within any legal definition of indecent images of children, and, given this, it is important to stress that collections of photographs of children per se are not in themselves indicative of anything inappropriate. It is the context of the photographs, and the way in which they are organised that is important.

> **Note**
> The statutory position is that, by virtue of section 1(1) of the Protection of Children Act 1978 (UK), it is an offence, in essence, to take or make an indecent photograph or pseudo-photograph of a child, or to distribute or show such photographs, or to possess such photographs with a view to their being distributed or shown, or to publish an advertisement conveying that the advertiser distributes or shows such photographs or intends to do so.

References

Akdeniz Y. The regulation of pornography and child pornography on the internet. *JILT*. 1997. www.2warwick.ac.uk/fac/soc/law/elj/jilt/1997_1/akdeniz1/

COPINE: www.copine.ie/

International Telecommunication Union: www.itu.int/ITU-D/ict/statistics/

Nielsen//NetRatings: www.nielsen-netratings.com/

Taylor M, Holland G, Quale E. Typology of paedophile picture collections. *Police Journal*. **74**(2): 97–107; 2001.

World Gazetteer: www.world-gazetteer.com/

Section Three conclusion

> We might conclude that rather than criminalising such activities in relation to the new technologies we should see them as a child protection issue, both for the victims in child abuse images and also for those victimised by a largely unregulated environment. (Quayle and Taylor, in press)

The Internet is a wonderful phenomenon; but it is open to misuse and users of any age can be vulnerable and fall prey to the unscrupulous abuser. It has sadly become a medium which is saturated with immoral and very often illegal sexually explicit material; a major concern as, for many young people, it is also a totally private world, where they feel at a distance from reality, anonymous and safe.

For parents

Consider for a moment how you prevent a baby falling from a child-restraining car seat the first time you use one? The answer is simple: you learn how to fasten them by using the safety straps. In other words, you learn how the safety features of the seat work.

Consider now how you prevent a young person falling victim to sexual abuse via the Internet? The answer again is simple. You learn how the parental controls and online safety features work and can be used. In other words, you learn how safety features of the Internet work.

You do not need a degree in computing to understand how the Internet, and in particular 'chat rooms', work in order to protect your child while online. Educational and advisory information describing the safe use of chat rooms and how they operate is commonly available from sources such as your ISP (Internet Service Provider). In addition, many children's charities and concerned authors have produced books or leaflets, available in shops and libraries, which outline the rudiments of safe Internet usage and communication for children and young people. If at present you do not have Internet access at home and your children are using the Internet at school or at Internet cafés, it may be advantageous to research a number of ISPs and establish what types of protection they provide for children before committing to a contract for online access at home. Most reputable ISPs will describe the parental controls they include in their package and will gladly explain how they work.

If your child is actively utilising the Internet and you have little knowledge about the nature or content of their usage, attempt to become more engaged in their 'Internet time'. By showing a greater interest in their online associates or 'keypals' and their general online activities, your child may feel more comfortable in sharing with you details of their contacts and the nature of the communication exchanged. In addition, encouraging your child to make more use of the Internet, thereby broadening their horizons, may increase the amount of Internet activity that your child 'allows' you to become involved in. This, in turn, may assist you in monitoring the level of activity in which your child engages and also give you the opportunity to identify the frequency and the date and times of communication with any regular 'contacts'.

Close supervision is always advisable when it comes to using the Internet, but as children grow older, it is not always possible to enforce such rules and young people will often access the Internet and 'chat' at all times of the day and night and with whom they choose. Faced with this situation, parents and carers need to monitor their child's behaviour and note any changes in behaviour which could be attributed to being groomed or abused. Parents and carers must be prepared to become a little intrusive and scrutinise the way in which their child uses computers.

For partners or associates

Be mindful that your partner, male or female, maybe a silent cyber-abuser.

Your partner may not harbour any intention to meet and then sexually abuse a child – he may solely wish to make contact with a child and maintain a cyber child-sex relationship which may fulfil his sexual and emotional needs. This may appear innocent enough, but the continual grooming, humiliation, emotional torment and negative effect upon the child victim's self-esteem could bring to a child victim untold and long-lasting psychological damage.

Although difficult to believe, your partner or spouse could be silently abusing your child through the Internet or mobile phone communication. If other behaviour by your partner or spouse has caused you concern, then it is important to monitor all activity including your partner's interest and scale of involvement in online activity; particularly if your partner is not your child's parent and is actively engaged in accessing the Internet with your child.

It has been known for male partners/husbands to maintain an apparently 'normal' relationship with their wife and children for many years, while silently abusing other children via the Internet. For such abusers, it is not uncommon for them to have amassed a large number of child contacts, networked abusers and a vast quantity of sexually abusive images of children which he will constantly trade with other abusers.

Common behaviours displayed by a partner or spouse silently abusing via the Internet:

- maintains, without good reason, a separate Internet account from the rest of the family
- purchases, without good reason, a second computer or mobile computer (laptop)
- accesses the Internet at unsociable hours or when you or the children are not at home
- remains in a locked room while accessing the Internet or enforces a 'closed door' practice having demanded isolation

- maintains a private 'compartment' on the family's computer hard drive where hidden information may be kept
- keeps a second hard drive, claiming it to be a spare and storing the 'spare' in an unknown or secure place
- frequently changes the main and 'spare' hard drive
- keeps a notebook or address book either secretly or accessible to the family but with the contents appearing to be written in code, or has a document or spreadsheet that is password protected and will not divulge its contents to you.

Be aware, also, that a partner or spouse may act in many of the ways above solely to hide his or her activity of engaging in seemingly harmless, legal adult cyber-sex with one or more individuals.

References

Quayle and Taylor. In press. www.innovationlaw.org/userfiles/page_attachments/ Library/1/Quayle_1223740.ppt.

Section Four

Action – by you and by others

12

Exercise plan – risk assessment

The ethos of this guide is simply to provide parents, child-carers and professionals with the knowledge, and therefore the opportunity, to accomplish for themselves the surety that their child, children, or children for whom they have responsibility, are protected from abusers; or to identify abuse and end it.

It is not sufficient merely to read this guide once and consider yourself adequately knowledgeable to identify a targeting would-be abuser; or consider yourself appropriately skilled to identify the many symptoms of abuse if displayed.

> This is a working guide designed to create and raise awareness in parents, child-carers and professionals to the existence of a potential abuser.

Whatever your personal circumstance, if you have children of your own or have access to children, you can become the focus point of a targeting paedophile that will use you as a conduit leading him to his chosen future victim. You may well, at this very moment, be that conduit.

If you regularly refresh your memory as to the common traits and behavioural patterns of active predatory paedophiles you greatly increase your chances of identifying such traits and patterns, should you or your family become a paedophile's target.

To assist in identifying a potential abuser, consider using the checklists below whenever a 'new' person enters your life, or a current contact behaves in such a way as to cause you concern. Copy the checklists, use them and store them in a safe place. Record times, dates and actions that appear to you to be inappropriate as well as actions, which in themselves appear harmless, but when carried out in conjunction with other actions, become concerning. Remember that a 'new' person could be a new partner, associate of your established partner, a neighbour, work colleague who imposes him or herself upon your home life, a parent of your child's new-found friend; anyone in fact whom you do not know and who may have contact with your child.

Tick off the specified characteristics and behaviours if and when identified. This will help to build a profile of the potential abuser. Do not forget that identifying in a man just *one or two* detailed characteristics and behaviours does not prove that he is abusing or has the potential to abuse children. Regular display, however, of quite a number of such characteristics and behaviours should arouse concern and appropriate action should be taken.

Log of concerning events

Copy or use this form, or make use of a diary, to record all known events which cause you concern. A detailed and dated record will assist you, social services and the police with any assessment, recommendations or investigation that may be required.

Date	Description of incident	Personal perspective

Record of identifiable characteristics and behaviour

By referring to Section One of this guide, making tentative enquires and asking subtle questions, monitor the actions of a person about whom you have concerns and mark this checklist of recognisable characteristics and behaviour when identified.

Characteristics and behaviour	✓	Notes
Abnormally interested in children		
Primary sexual arousal/interest is solely directed towards children		
Primary sexual arousal/interest becomes diverted from adults towards children		
Initial focus/attention towards children involves impulsive acts		
Suffers from stress/depression		
Appears hyperactive/nervous or anxious		
Recent increase in alcohol/ substance abuse causing uninhibited sexualised behaviour towards children		
History of short romantic common-law relationships		
Has strong cognitive distortions (twists accounts of incidents to suit his needs)		
Minimises blameworthy events or suspicious behaviour		
Is well ordered and precise		
Fails to develop good relationships with peers		
Claims offence was 'totally out of character' and a 'one-off' occurrence		

Characteristics and behaviour	✓	*Notes*
Lives alone or with both parents or mother		
His friends are of a similar, like-minded nature		
Circulates/shares your family and personal details with others		
Possesses an unusually large number of images of children (not necessary indecent)		
Continuously/regularly pays attention to children of a specific gender, age, and physical description		
Pays particular attention to vulnerable children		
Pays particular attention to physically and/or mentally handicapped children		
Displays regular behaviour which brings him into contact with children		
Uses certain descriptive words or phrases which may indicate an unhealthy liking for children		
Has a history of association with youth groups		
Has unexplained reasons for changes in employment		
Has numerous previous jobs which involved association with children		
Has gained various unconnected qualifications, which aid access to children		
Follows a clear pattern of behaviour in making contact with children		

Characteristics and behaviour	✓	Notes
Is a youth leader or plays official role in a children's organisation		
By words and actions, continuously portrays himself as a nice man		
Initially, pays great attention to the parent/s or guardians and ignores the targeted child		
Pays particular attention to one specific child		
Undesirably attaches himself to one parent to gain access to a child or a group of children		
Is attentive to children and invests a great deal of time in making them feel special		
Will seek to display his actions as normal, convincing the naive parent and child all is well		
Possesses in his home material/music/games that appeal to children – not befitting an adult		
Exposes children to pornography on an escalating scale to lower inhibitions		
Drives a wedge between parent and child – adopting a pseudo-parental role		
Is clearly happiest when in the company of children and enjoys photographing them		
Goes to great lengths to be alone with the targeted child		
Puts himself out and appears to be a martyr		
Has a history of indecent exposure convictions		

Characteristics and behaviour	✓	Notes
Possesses/views indecent images of children – claiming that this is his only perversion		
Uses his own children to make contact with other children and parents or carers		
Associates with parents of disabled children when he clearly has none		
Claims not to like children or requests that children are kept at a distance; later, becomes greatly involved with children		
Discloses early in relationship his cautions or convictions for child sex abuse, claiming to be innocent		
Falsely claims to be a parent or having responsibility for other children		
Becomes indispensable to the parent/carer		

13

Guiding your child through disclosure

Disclosure of abuse

It would be a devastating occurrence for any loving and caring parent or carer to discover that his or her child is suffering or has suffered any form of abuse. It would be easy and understandable for a parent or carer to become enraged, scream and shout and threaten to kill the abuser. This behaviour, however, will not help your child. If your child begins to tell you about being the victim of abuse, particularly sexual abuse, consider how difficult and frightening it must be for your child to do so. If you think that your child has not disclosed all there is to tell, do not pressurise your child to disclose further. A more detailed or a more explanatory disclosure may well follow at a later date, when your child is satisfied that he or she is being believed and his or her account of the events is being taken seriously.

Remember that the abuser may well have undermined your parental role and attempted to reduce your child's liking and love for you as well as his or her trust in you. Take time rebuilding these essential factors and do not rush or pressurise your child into anything.

The age of your child and the relationship between your child and the abuser may well determine his or her view on reporting the matter to the police or social services. A young child will not have any say in the matter, as the decision is solely that of the parent/carer. However, an older child, e.g. a 15-year-old male, may just want the abuse to stop and not involve the authorities. Simply not sending him to 'Granddad's' on a Saturday afternoon will end the 15-year-old's torment.

Once a disclosure of abuse has been made, for the physical and psychological benefit of your child, do not allow your child in the company of the alleged abuser, even if supervised.

There is no right and wrong answer in deciding whether to report the matter or not. It is for the victim and parents/carers to decide what is best for the victim.

Consideration must be given, however, to the fact that if the abuser is not brought to the attention of the police or social services, he may continue to abuse other children. He may well be abusing or grooming other children at the very moment you decide not to involve the authorities. It is not impossible, however, to inform the police or social services about the abuser and his activities without making a full complaint. This allows the authorities to monitor the abuser, obstruct his grooming activities and prevent further abuse. In addition, the authorities can identify other children he may be abusing.

Parents

If your child begins to describe events, or details of a person whom he or she fears, the following should be considered.

- Take your child to a familiar and safe location and be willing to re-locate and be quick to respond if the chosen location is identified by your child as the place where the abuse occurred.
- Arrange for peace and quiet by having siblings, other adults and pets away from the chosen location. Do not allow other people to become involved. At this stage, disclosure details of the abuser may not be given and, should the abuser walk in on your discussion, this could well disrupt your child's account and full disclosure may never happen.
- Give your child your complete and utter attention – affirming to them that you are absorbing all that is said.
- Do not make assumptions. Listen and accept what is said.
- Encourage your child to talk openly and fully, but do not pressurise or persist for more information or claim that more must have happened. Do not become part of your child's problem by dramatising the events, embellishing the events or making suggestions as to what else may have happened. Simply accept from your child what is said at that time, as further disclosure may follow.
- It is rare that children lie about abuse. Certain issues will stand out as being obviously concerning, such as a five-year-old girl describing adult male genitalia or other sexual matters not normally known by a child of such an age.
- Explain to your child that you believe everything that has been said, even if certain or all points raised appear unbelievable; your child may well be suffering from shock as a result of experiencing, for the first time, talking with you about sexual matters and abuse. He or she may be confused and has spoken hurriedly and without conscious effort to structure the account. Be aware that more precise chronological details and explanations can be obtained once the initial shock is over and the child has calmed. This may take a number of days.
- Make it clear, firmly, that he or she has not misbehaved or is in any way responsible for the events that have occurred. The blame lies with the abuser.
- Emphasise the fact that whatever the abuser has said or threatened, it will not be true. If the abuser has instilled fear into your child by violence, dispel any fears that your child may have by explaining that the abuser will no longer be able to make contact with your child and that your child will be left alone.
- Give praise to your child for being brave and speaking out about the abuse. Explain that you are aware of how difficult speaking about the events must be and that you are thankful that your child chose you to speak to. Although difficult, if asked, do not give your promise that you and your child will keep this matter a secret. For the sake of other children at least, authorities must be made aware of the abuser.
- If your child's character had noticeably changed leading up to the disclosure and your child had been misbehaving, playing truant, or is depressed or angry, explain that you hold no ill feeling about these matters and pay little attention to them.
- Make a sincere promise to your child that the abuse will stop. Discussion concerning disclosure to the authorities may have to be held later. A more thorough discussion with your child at a later time may benefit your child, but be mindful that with certain sexual abuse offences, forensic evidence may be lost if disclosure and physical examination is delayed.
- It is imperative to constantly support your child from the moment a disclosure is made. A child who has built up the strength to disclose an abusive sexual

act to you will have come a long way in his or her mind. If the support needed is lacking, then the child may well withdraw and refuse to divulge further details or refrain from discussing the issue with professionals if reported.

- Inform the police or social services without delay. If the reporting of the child's disclosure to the authorities is immediate, then you are reaffirming to the child that you believe the account that he or she has given. You are also providing greater protection for the child and will be assisting the authorities in apprehending the abuser before further harm can be caused to other children.

Teachers and carers

If a child begins to describe events, or details of a person whom he or she fears, these additional points should also be considered.

- Protect the child from other children and other adults who don't need to know, but do notify a member of staff (ideally an education welfare officer if available) of the situation. Do not immediately contact the parents or guardians as one or both of these people could be the abuser.
- Be aware of your organisation's policy on disclosure – you may need to be in the company of another professional to listen to a child talk on such matters, or refrain from engaging with the child and seek professional help. The latter is not ideal as the child concerned clearly feels that he or she can confide in you and you should make every effort to capitalise on his or her confidence for the greater benefit of the child.
- You are the first witness. Try to remember everything that is said. Your evidence could assist the police and social services in any future investigation. Do not sit in front of the child and write down what the child says verbatim. This may well dissuade the child from speaking freely, so avoid writing as the child talks. Attempt to memorise all the child says and make notes after the event as soon as is practicable.
- Inform the child that either or both social services and the police will be informed. Do not call social services and the police without the child being aware. To be suddenly confronted with an unknown adult, particularly one in uniform, could distress and frighten the child – particularly if the child has been groomed in such a way that he or she has an avid fear of police or social service officialdom. In addition, the offender may be an individual who, during the grooming and offending process, has worn a uniform of a certain type so as to appear as an authoritative figure.
- If possible, keep the child with you or with another staff member in a safe and secure place. You have no legal power to restrain or detain the child in such circumstances, but having the child with you until police officers or social service workers arrive and 'take charge' can only be a good thing.

Details required and questions parents and teachers should consider asking

It is important to identify and validate as much information as possible concerning the victim and the occurrence. Therefore, all knowledge of the victim and circumstances known by the person receiving the complaint, and/or informing police or social services, should be documented. In addition, if it were felt that the child is capable and willing to answer questions, careful and considerate questioning should be considered.

The following compilation of known details and answers would assist the police, social services and other agencies greatly in formulating an immediate reaction plan.

Safety measures

- Current location and current safety level of child.
- Any physical injuries that require immediate hospital or other medical treatment.
- Any apparent psychological concerns.
- Is the suspected abuser nearby?
- Is there a likelihood of having imminent contact with the suspected abuser?
- Are any other children at immediate and significant risk from the suspected abuser?

Personal details

- Full identity and contact details of the person reporting.
- Full identity and contact details of the person receiving complaint (if different).
- Full identity details of the victim (name, sex, date of birth, home address, telephone numbers, etc.).
- Full identity details of the victim's family members (natural, adoptive or fostered).
- Is there any history of social services involvement?
- Any information concerning court orders.
- Details of the victim's school and general practitioner.
- Any information concerning 'special needs'.

Occurrence details

- Nature of the incident (single or recurring happening, prolonged episode).
- Person alleged to be responsible.
- Location of the incident.
- Details and locations of any witnesses.
- Are weapons involved?
- Description of the demeanour displayed by victim, witnesses or perpetrator.
- Does any person involved (victim, witnesses or perpetrators) seem to be under the influence of alcohol or drugs?

> If you become aware of child abuse, in any form, occurring to any child, it is imperative to inform the police or social services' Child Protection Units.

14

Police and social services procedures

Initial disclosure

- The notification to the authorities of a child's exposure to abuse, of any sort, can be made by the victim, by any other member of the public or any person from any professional agency. A child may choose to disclose his or her suffering of abuse by way of informing a parent, other relative, a teacher, a close school or family friend, medical staff at a local hospital or general practice surgery or by telephoning or e-mailing a children's charity organisation. Generally, children choose to either disclose to a person whom they feel most comfortable in speaking with and confiding in, or by contacting a child support organisation. The person selected by the child, to whom he or she wishes to disclose, should always inform the authorities of the disclosure in the first instance.
- Disclosure to the authorities will trigger a practised and well-proven procedure which is, generally, nationally consistent. Minor differences in the procedure between one authority locality and another or from one police force to another are often governed by geography, staff resources or specific requirements dependent upon local community issues. Such differences will be agreed between local professional agencies as policy or best practice.

Action by police and social services following an initial disclosure of abuse

Receipt of disclosure

Any police officer or police staff member or social services staff member can receive an initial disclosure. Such disclosures are to be forwarded without delay to the agency's own Child Protection Unit, where the disclosure will be recorded and subjected to continual review and assessment. Police forces across the country utilise various terms or acronyms for their child protection units. Some forces use: Child Abuse Investigation Team (CAIT) or Child Abuse Investigation Unit (CAIU). For the purposes of simplicity in this chapter, the police Child Protection Unit will be referred to as CAIT.

Social services departments (SSDs) across the country also utilise various names for their child protection offices. Again, for simplicity, one specific term will be used in this guide. Child Protection Department or CPD will be used when referring to social services child protection offices or staff.

Completion of referral form

Different agencies and localities will have established their own specific 'referral form' but the details contained therein will be the same. It will include details of the victim, the victim's family, other significant people in the victim's life, details of professionals previously involved with the victim, details of the perpetrator as in-depth as possible and a detailed outline of events leading to the disclosure. The referral will be housed in a secure location and updated with entries outlining all actions by CAIT or CPD and any other relevant information along with an account as to the progress of the investigation.

Sharing of information/strategy

Joint agency working, sharing information and strategy

CAIT and CPD will immediately share with each other details of the disclosure and any other information concerning the victim, the victim's family or perpetrator. They will discuss the current risks to the victim (if any), risks to other children, and support for family or friends as is required. CAIT and CPD team leaders or supervisors will create an agreed strategy for dealing with the victim in an expeditious fashion that is also in the victim's best interest. The strategy discussion will involve the consideration, planning and arranging of: the safety and well being of the victim, reducing risks, the CAIT (police) interview of the victim, housing/placement of the victim where required, and the arrest of the perpetrator if immediately necessary.

A child in need

Section 17(10) of the Children Act 1989 states that a child shall be taken to be in need if:

1   he is unlikely to achieve or maintain, or to have the opportunity of achieving or maintaining, a reasonable standard of health or development without the provision for him of services by a local authority under this part
2   his health or development is likely to be significantly impaired, or further impaired, without the provision of such services; or
3   he is disabled.

Early in the 'sharing of information' stage, a joint agency decision will be made by team leaders or supervisors, as to whether the child concerned is likely or not to be at risk of suffering significant harm. If it is evident that the child concerned is not at such a risk, both the police and SSD still have a responsibility should it be felt that the child is in need. The local authority, under Section 17 of the Children Act 1989, has a duty to safeguard and promote the welfare of children within their area by providing various services. Although police do not have a specific role with regards to children in need, if any police officer feels that a child is in such need then he or she should report their findings to the CAIT or CPD.

Criminal investigation and social services family intervention and support

Police and social services interview (of victim and abuser)

An interview of a child takes place after careful thought and planning by a multidisciplinary body and should be conducted without delay.

The nature of interview conducted by police will depend upon the type of abuse alleged and the current age of the victim. Victims of physical, emotional and neglect-type abuse (who are *15* years or younger at the time of the allegation) and victims of sexual abuse (who are *16* years or younger at the time of the allegation) will be offered the opportunity to disclose the evidence of the abuse, when it is felt necessary, by way of police video-recorded interview. In every case, the interviews conducted will follow a strict pattern: a specially developed pattern of practice to ensure the psychological well being of the victim.

Most police forces have developed and maintain victim interview rooms that are located some distance from police stations. The interview rooms are usually decorated and furnished characteristically like a common domestic lounge and are located within a property resembling a typical house or flat. Microphones and cameras are located within the interview room and these are overt as it is vital that the victim is aware that he or she is being recorded both audibly and visually. The interview is carried out with every effort to make the victim feel relaxed and comfortable, thus helping to reduce the level of stress and anxiety the child may feel.

The whole idea of video-recording a victim's interview is to obtain as much detailed evidence as is possible including the body language, facial expressions and reactions of the child when asked questions by the interviewing officer, and while disclosing evidence. The video can be played in court allowing the victim freedom from giving evidence in front of a judge, jury and, most importantly, the perpetrator.

The necessity for an immediate medical examination by a suitably qualified doctor – for both medical and evidential purposes

It is important, for both the child victim and the police, that the injured or abused child receives an examination by a suitably qualified doctor, namely a paediatrician. This is to ascertain the full extent of the nature of the abuse or injury and to ensure that the child receives the correct treatment; it is also to secure any available forensic evidence. It is also important that any signs of injury or evidence of such injury is documented by the paediatrician and photographed by a suitably qualified photographer, namely a police crime scene investigator.

On occasions, it is necessary for such examinations and photographing to take place with some degree of expediency. This is often due to the fact that at the time a disclosure is made by a child, outlining a form of sexual or physical abuse, it is not always known if the case will lead to a criminal prosecution. However, all aspects of forensic and occurrence-evidence gathering should be commenced, provided that the child victim is not caused any unnecessary distress and it is in the child's best interest.

Some physical forensic evidence pertaining to sexual or physical abuse does not remain available for a protracted period of time. Semen, blood, saliva or skin tissue can be deliberately, accidentally or naturally washed away from certain body areas within hours or even minutes of an incident of abuse taking place. Skin damage, bruising and in particular finger-marks can change appearance or even disappear within hours of being caused, and it is therefore necessary for a medical examination and photographing to take place as soon as is practicable to secure evidence samples and visual images.

Necessity to arrest immediately

If the child victim is at a place of safety or at a location where he or she is free from the likelihood of being confronted by the perpetrator, one could argue that arrest is not urgent and other matters such as securing evidence, victim interview and research into possible other victims should take precedence. In many cases this is so.

In others, however, particularly when the most recent or only abuse incident occurred within a short period of time, arrest of the perpetrator is vital in securing possible physical evidence by seizing clothing, bedding and other articles for forensic examination at a later date. The perpetrator can also be examined and samples of blood or semen obtained to identify the perpetrator's DNA profile.

In cases where a victim has made an allegation against a person, and that person is not likely to come into contact with the victim, but has or possibly has contact with other children, a decision to arrest immediately to safeguard the 'other' children may well be made.

Criminal investigation

The criminal investigation commences the moment a referral or an allegation is made to the police. Obviously, not all referrals or allegations result in a criminal investigation by virtue of being either false, a misunderstanding of the initial disclosure or being deemed to be a case of a child in need, as opposed to child abuse.

Once established that the case is that of child abuse, the criminal investigation continues and arrangements for the interviewing of the child victim are made. In accordance with Home Office guidelines, all children under the age of 16 years are interviewed by way of video-interview.

Witnesses will also be video-interviewed if under the age of 16 or considered vulnerable.

If evidence is obtained from the video-interview, it will be added to the evidence obtained from witnesses and forensic examination. The police and staff of the Crown Prosecution Services (CPS) will then assess the evidence and a decision will be made by the CPS as to whether sufficient evidence exists to go ahead with criminal proceedings.

Social services allocation of social worker and case assessment

Upon receipt of a referral, and following an ensuing strategy, a suitably qualified social worker employed by the local authority SSD will be allocated to the child, both or either of the parents or the family as a whole, as is necessary. The case will be subject to what is known as 'a Section 17 investigation'. The investigation will determine if the case warrants monitoring by a Case Conference Committee. If so, a multi-agency case conference will be held, bringing professionals from a variety of agencies together, to view the case details and dictate initial action to be taken to safeguard children. In cases where concern for a child's welfare is ongoing, personnel from all agencies able to offer support, guidance and where needed control will meet regularly to ascertain the current situation regarding the child's general welfare. Persons from the relevant agencies are known as the Case Conference Committee, within which is a 'core group' of professionals who will work directly with the child, the parents or the family.

During these conferences, a number of factors are discussed; these can range from details of all persons having involvement with the child, risk indicators or the positive or negative issues impacting upon the child's psychological and physical development. On conclusion of a case conference, an action plan is created to address all issues raised.

Note

It is at such joint-agency Case Conferences that decisions are made as to whether a child's name should appear, continue to appear or be removed from the 'at-risk register'. Such decisions are only made with the agreement of all persons concerned.

The Child Protection Register

All social services departments with Great Britain are duty bound to maintain Child Protection Registers. The Register, which is confidential, is a list of children who reside within the local authority area and are considered to be at risk of significant harm. The local authority, having identified such a child, must protect the child by way of a 'child protection plan', the contents of which are actions set to reduce the risk of such harm. The Case Conference Committee, Register and plan help to coordinate and assist all those persons involved with a child in his or her protection.

Victim Support and counselling

Victim Support is a self-funding, charity-based organisation, which relies heavily upon its volunteer staff to give both their time and effort in supporting victims. Trained individuals, often ex-police officers and counsellors who offer advice and counselling services, staff the agency.

Police investigators and social service workers are familiar with Victim Support and other organisations and individuals who offer counselling and support to both the victim and the victim's family members.

Police and social services powers

Lawful power given to the police to remove or detain a child

Police Protection Powers

A lawful power under Section 46 of the Children Act 1989 allows a constable who has reasonable cause to believe that a child would otherwise be likely to suffer significant harm to:

- remove a child to suitable accommodation and keep her or him there
- take such steps as are reasonable to ensure that the child's removal from any hospital, or other place, in which she or he is then being accommodated, is prevented.

Definition of a 'place of safety' or 'suitable accommodation'

Having exercised Police Protection Powers, the officers concerned must take the child(ren) to a place of safety such as the local social services office, the home of a suitable temporary foster carer or children's home. The child(ren) will remain at this location until such a time as either:

- full-time foster carers are granted custody of the child(ren) by a court
- suitable family members (not parents) are granted custody of the child(ren) by a court
- the parents are able to provide such necessary care.

Police officers should only take a child or children under Police Protection Powers to a police station in extreme cases; usually when all other avenues for accommodation have been explored but failed. If this is the case, children should only be kept at a police station for the minimum of time required.

Example 1

Uniformed police officers are instructed to attend at the residential home address of the Smith family following information received that the parents regularly drink heavily and argue. The arguments regularly escalate to domestic violence occurring between the parents, which has been witnessed by both the family's two children, aged six and seven years, and neighbours. Upon arrival, the officers find the parents highly inebriated and unable to satisfactorily supervise the children in their care.

The children are not at a place of safety and are at risk of significant harm. Neither suitable family members nor suitable friends can be found to take charge of the children and so measures must be taken by the officers attending to provide safety for the children. In this case, the officers are wholly justified in taking the children into police custody, removing them from the family home and taking them to a place of safety.

Example 2

Police officers execute a search warrant at an address known to be occupied by a male drug user and dealer. Upon entry, officers find at the address the known male and his female partner. His female partner has a two-year-old daughter who was fathered by another male. No drugs were located, but the living area was littered with drug-taking paraphernalia (hypodermic needles, pieces of glass and razor blades). The daughter was seen walking freely among the paraphernalia. At the same time, the adults were found to be under the influence of drugs but were not beyond the ability to supervise the child; however, the environment was wholly unsuitable for the child and she remained at significant risk of harm if she continued to remain at the address. The adults were unable to nominate any other suitable adults to provide care for the child and therefore officers took the child into police custody, taking her to a suitable place of safety.

Example 3

Hospital staff, working at an accident and emergency unit, are presented with a heavily bruised, nine-month-old male child who is also suffering with a broken arm. The child was brought to the unit by a woman claiming to be the boy's mother. She provides an unlikely account for the injuries. Following a medical examination, medical staff inform the police of the circumstances and their concerns. Uniformed police attend the unit as a matter of urgency and speak with the woman purporting to be the mother. She immediately attempts to remove the child from the unit with the intention of leaving the hospital. Both the medical staff and police officers believe that the injuries may have been caused deliberately and that, if left alone with the woman, the child would be at risk of significant harm. The child is also in need of immediate and continued medical attention. The officers in this case are legally justified and have a duty to act by way of taking the child into police custody and maintaining his presence at the hospital which is a suitable place of safety and where he can receive the necessary treatment.

Power given to local departments of social services to remove or detain a child

Emergency Protection Order

This is a lawful order under Section 44 of the Children Act 1989, which can be obtained from a magistrate if the magistrate is satisfied that that there is reasonable cause to believe that a child is likely to suffer significant harm if:

- the child is not removed to safe accommodation or
- the child does not remain in the place in which he or she is then being accommodated.

A separate lawful order under Section 47 of the Children Act 1989 can also be obtained if enquiries are being frustrated by access to the child being unreasonably refused to a person authorised to seek access, and the applicant has reasonable cause to believe that access is needed as a matter of urgency.

An Emergency Protection Order gives authority to remove a child, and places the child under the protection of the applicant for a maximum period of eight days, with a possible extension for a further seven days.

Example 1

A 20-year-old female, known to the department of social services following an historic suicide attempt and continued drug misuse, becomes pregnant and intends to keep the child. The child is born and it is necessary to wean the child from an addiction of heroin. Constant contact with mother and child shows that

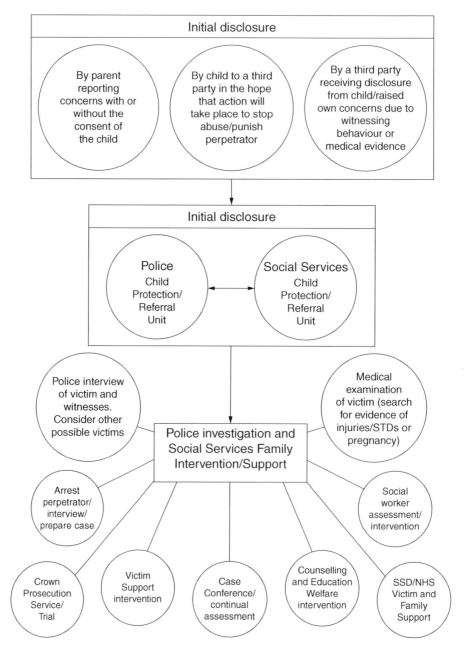

Figure 14.1 Joint agency working – a general description of initial action by police and social services.

the mother continues to misuse heroin and often places herself and her child at risk of harm, by way of associating with drug users (using drugs in the mother's accommodation in the company of the child) and also by way of bringing to the home numerous men who are clients for prostitution. Both the drug users and male clients are often heavily intoxicated by either drink or drugs, and arguments and violence have occurred in the presence of the child. After repeated warnings and constant offers of support, the mother refuses to change her ways. Generally, the mother's direct care for the child is reasonable, but her behaviour, associations and profession places her child at risk of significant harm. Following assessments and a joint-agency conference, the decision was made to remove the child to a place of safety.

In this case, social services staff are correct in applying for an Emergency Protection Order and a magistrate is wholly justified in issuing such an order.

Example 2

A child attends her local school as normal. Teaching staff notice specific bruising to her shoulders, neck and face. They briefly speak with the child and she reveals that 'Daddy did it'. Staff at the school inform the local department of social services. A joint agency meeting is held between the SSD, police and education welfare and a decision is made to speak with the child's mother and interview/ arrest the father. If the father is to be released following a police interview, it is necessary to ascertain if he would reside elsewhere for the interim period, therefore not posing a risk of physical harm to the child. If mother and father both deny that the father is responsible and/or do not agree to residing separately, the child is likely to be at risk of significant harm.

In this case, social services staff would be wholly justified in seeking an Emergency Protection Order and removing the child from the parents' care. *See* Figure 14.1.

Victoria Climbié – *The Laming Report* and *Every Child Matters*

The Secretary of State for Health, under Section 81 of the Children Act 1989 and under Section 84 of the NHS Act 1997, and the Secretary of State for the Home Department, under Section 49 of the Police Act 1996, appointed Lord Laming to conduct an inquiry into the circumstances surrounding the death of Victoria Climbié, which occurred in February 2000.

In 2003, Lord Laming's report into the inquiry, which included his findings and recommendations, was published (Victoria Climbié Inquiry 2003). At the same time, the Government published a green paper called *Every Child Matters* (HM Treasury 2003). This publication was based on original plans which were set to enhance child protection services by concentrating on four specific issues:

- increasing the focus on supporting families and carers – the critical influence on children's lives
- ensuring necessary intervention takes place before children reach crisis point and protecting children from falling through the net

- addressing the underlying problems identified in the report into the death of Victoria Climbié – weak accountability and poor integration
- ensuring that people working with children are valued, rewarded and trained.

In 2004, the Government published *Every Child Matters: change for children* (DfES 2004b), *Every Child Matters: the next steps* (DfES 2004a), and the Children Act 2004. These three publications create a legislative structure which leads towards improved and accessible services, whose role it is to support and focus upon the needs of children, young people and families.

Every Child Matters calls for organisations involved with the care of children, young persons and families to work together in new ways, to readily share information, to protect children and young persons from harm, and to help them develop and achieve their potential in life.

References

Department for Education and Skills (DfES). *Every Child Matters: change for children.* London: Department for Education and Skills; 2004a.
Department for Education and Skills (DfES). *Every Child Matters: the next steps.* London: Department for Education and Skills; 2004b.
HM Treasury. *Every Child Matters.* London: The Stationery Office; 2003
Victoria Climbié Inquiry. *The Laming Report.* 2003. www.nationalarchives.gov.uk/ERO/records/vc/1/1/index.htm

15

Sexual offences – the law

> Sex Offenders Act 1997
> Sexual Offences Act 2000
> Criminal Justice and Court Services Act 2000
> Sexual Offences Act 2003

In September 1997, the Sex Offenders Act came into force introducing the Sex Offenders Register. Part 1 of the Sex Offenders Act 1997 required persons who were convicted or cautioned (or otherwise required to do so) for relevant sex offences to notify the police of their name, date of birth, address and any subsequent changes to them.

The Sex Offenders Act 1997 had a number of faults and legal loopholes, which have been overcome by changes to the legislation. In 2002, the Government proposed a white paper, *Protecting the Public*, outlining new legislation, which became the Sexual Offences Act 2003.

This new Act has two parts. Part One of the Act clarifies sexual offences and outlines the revisions and amendments that strengthen the law concerning sexual offending.

Part Two details a revised system of sex offenders' registration, which replaces many of the provisions of the Sex Offenders Act 1997. Also included in Part Two of the Act are provisions for the service of sex offending and risk of harm, preventative orders. These orders are made under civil law, but applied for by police or other agencies at criminal courts. The orders, once served and imposed, restrict the actions and movements of sex offenders or other persons who have been assessed as posing a risk of serious sexual harm to others.

> **Note**
> Below is a brief overview of selected sections and information from the Act that is most relevant to persons convicted of sex offences, or otherwise meeting the criteria for sex offender registration. Reference should be made to the Act in full for all provisions stipulated by statute.

Persons becoming subject to Notification Order requirements

1 A person is subject to the notification requirements of this Part for the period set out in section 82 (the notification periods as detailed below) if:
   a   he is convicted of an offence listed in Schedule 3 (as detailed below)
   b   he is found not guilty of such an offence by reason of insanity

    c he is found to be under a disability and to have done the act charged against him in respect of such an offence; or

    d in England and Wales or Northern Ireland, he is cautioned in respect of such an offence.

2 A person for the time being subject to the notification requirements of this Part is referred to in this Part as a 'relevant offender'. (Crown Copyright)

Schedule 3 offences

1 An offence under section 1 of the Sexual Offences Act 1956 (c. 69) (rape).

2 An offence under section 5 of that Act (intercourse with girl under 13).

3 An offence under section 6 of that Act (intercourse with girl under 16), if the offender was 20 or over.

4 An offence under section 10 of that Act (incest by a man), if the victim or (as the case may be) other party was under 18.

5 An offence under section 12 of that Act (buggery) if:

    a the offender was 20 or over, and

    b the victim or (as the case may be) other party was under 18.

6 An offence under section 13 of that Act (indecency between men) if:

    a the offender was 20 or over, and

    b the victim or (as the case may be) other party was under 18.

7 An offence under section 14 of that Act (indecent assault on a woman) if:

    a the victim or (as the case may be) other party was under 18, or

    b the offender, in respect of the offence or finding, is or has been:

        i   sentenced to imprisonment for a term of at least 30 months; or

        ii admitted to a hospital subject to a restriction order.

8 An offence under section 15 of that Act (indecent assault on a man) if:

    a the victim or (as the case may be) other party was under 18, or

    b the offender, in respect of the offence or finding, is or has been:

        i   sentenced to imprisonment for a term of at least 30 months; or

        ii admitted to a hospital subject to a restriction order.

9 An offence under section 16 of that Act (assault with intent to commit buggery), if the victim or (as the case may be) other party was under 18.

10 An offence under section 28 of that Act (causing or encouraging the prostitution of, intercourse with or indecent assault on girl under 16).

11 An offence under section 1 of the Indecency with Children Act 1960 (c. 33) (indecent conduct towards young child).

12 An offence under section 54 of the Criminal Law Act 1977 (c. 45) (inciting girl under 16 to have incestuous sexual intercourse).

13 An offence under section 1 of the Protection of Children Act 1978 (c. 37) (indecent photographs of children), if the indecent photographs or pseudo-photographs showed persons under 16 and:

    a the conviction, finding or caution was before the commencement of this Part, or

    b the offender:

        i   was 18 or over, or

        ii is sentenced in respect of the offence to imprisonment for a term of at least 12 months.

14 An offence under section 170 of the Customs and Excise Management Act 1979 (c. 2) (penalty for fraudulent evasion of duty, etc.) in relation to goods prohibited to be imported under section 42 of the Customs Consolidation Act 1876 (c. 36) (indecent or obscene articles), if the prohibited goods included indecent photographs of persons under 16 and:

    a the conviction, finding or caution was before the commencement of this Part, or

    b the offender:

       i was 18 or over, or

       ii is sentenced in respect of the offence to imprisonment for a term of at least 12 months.

15 An offence under section 160 of the Criminal Justice Act 1988 (c. 33) (possession of indecent photographs of a child), if the indecent photographs or pseudo-photographs showed persons under 16 and:

    a the conviction, finding or caution was before the commencement of this Part, or

    b the offender:

       i was 18 or over, or

       ii is sentenced in respect of the offence to imprisonment for a term of at least 12 months.

16 An offence under section 3 of the Sexual Offences (Amendment) Act 2000 (c. 44) (abuse of position of trust), if the offender was 20 or over.

17 An offence under section 1 or 2 of this Act (rape, assault by penetration).

18 An offence under section 3 of this Act (sexual assault) if:

    a where the offender was under 18, he is or has been sentenced, in respect of the offence, to imprisonment for a term of at least 12 months

    b in any other case:

       i the victim was under 18, or

       ii the offender, in respect of the offence or finding, is or has been:

          a sentenced to a term of imprisonment

          b detained in a hospital, or

          c made the subject of a community sentence of at least 12 months.

19 An offence under any of sections 4 to 6 of this Act (causing sexual activity without consent, rape of a child under 13, assault of a child under 13 by penetration).

20 An offence under section 7 of this Act (sexual assault of a child under 13) if the offender:

    a was 18 or over, or

    b is or has been sentenced in respect of the offence to imprisonment for a term of at least 12 months.

21 An offence under any of sections 8 to 12 of this Act (causing or inciting a child under 13 to engage in sexual activity, child sex offences committed by adults).

22 An offence under section 13 of this Act (child sex offences committed by children or young persons), if the offender is or has been sentenced, in respect of the offence, to imprisonment for a term of at least 12 months.

23 An offence under section 14 of this Act (arranging or facilitating the commission of a child sex offence) if the offender:

    a   was 18 or over, or

    b   is or has been sentenced, in respect of the offence, to imprisonment for a term of at least 12 months.

24   An offence under section 15 of this Act (meeting a child following sexual grooming, etc.).

25   An offence under any of sections 16 to 19 of this Act (abuse of a position of trust) if the offender, in respect of the offence, is or has been:

    a   sentenced to a term of imprisonment

    b   detained in a hospital, or

    c   made the subject of a community sentence of at least 12 months.

26   An offence under section 25 or 26 of this Act (familial child sex offences) if the offender:

    a   was 18 or over, or

    b   is or has been sentenced in respect of the offence to imprisonment for a term of at least 12 months.

27   An offence under any of sections 30 to 37 of this Act (offences against persons with a mental disorder impeding choice, inducements, etc., to persons with mental disorder).

28   An offence under any of sections 38 to 41 of this Act (care workers for persons with mental disorder) if:

    a   where the offender was under 18, he is or has been sentenced in respect of the offence to imprisonment for a term of at least 12 months

    b   in any other case, the offender, in respect of the offence or finding, is or has been:

       i   sentenced to a term of imprisonment,

       ii   detained in a hospital, or

       iii   made the subject of a community sentence of at least 12 months.

29   An offence under section 47 of this Act (paying for sexual services of a child) if the victim or (as the case may be) other party was under 16, and the offender:

    a   was 18 or over, or

    b   is or has been sentenced in respect of the offence to imprisonment for a term of at least 12 months.

30   An offence under section 61 of this Act (administering a substance with intent).

31   An offence under section 62 or 63 of this Act (committing an offence or trespassing, with intent to commit a sexual offence) if:

    a   where the offender was under 18, he is or has been sentenced in respect of the offence to imprisonment for a term of at least 12 months

    b   in any other case:

       i   the intended offence was an offence against a person under 18, or

       ii   the offender, in respect of the offence or finding, is or has been:

          a   sentenced to a term of imprisonment

          b   detained in a hospital, or

          c   made the subject of a community sentence of at least 12 months.

32   An offence under section 64 or 65 of this Act (sex with an adult relative) if:

    a   where the offender was under 18, he is or has been sentenced in respect of the offence to imprisonment for a term of at least 12 months

    b in any other case, the offender, in respect of the offence or finding, is or
has been:
      i sentenced to a term of imprisonment, or
      ii detained in a hospital.

33 An offence under section 66 of this Act (exposure) if:
    a where the offender was under 18, he is or has been sentenced in respect
of the offence to imprisonment for a term of at least 12 months
    b in any other case:
      i the victim was under 18, or
      ii the offender, in respect of the offence or finding, is or has been:
        a sentenced to a term of imprisonment
        b detained in a hospital, or
        c made the subject of a community sentence of at least 12 months.

34 An offence under section 67 of this Act (voyeurism) if:
    a where the offender was under 18, he is or has been sentenced in respect
of the offence to imprisonment for a term of at least 12 months
    b in any other case:
      i the victim was under 18, or
      ii the offender, in respect of the offence or finding, is or has been:
        a sentenced to a term of imprisonment
        b detained in a hospital, or
        c made the subject of a community sentence of at least 12 months.

35 An offence under section 69 or 70 of this Act (intercourse with an animal,
sexual penetration of a corpse) if:
    a where the offender was under 18, he is or has been sentenced in respect
of the offence to imprisonment for a term of at least 12 months
    b in any other case, the offender, in respect of the offence or finding, is or
has been:
      i sentenced to a term of imprisonment, or
      ii detained in a hospital.

Note

Schedule 3 offences differ for Scotland and Northern Ireland. Details
of the Act and all parts pertaining to 'relevant offences' can be obtained
from Her Majesty's Stationery Office website: www.legislation.hmso.gov.uk
(Crown Copyright).

Notification periods

Description of relevant offender	Notification period
A person who, in respect of the offence, is or has been sentenced to imprisonment for life or for a term of 30 months or more	An indefinite period beginning with the relevant date
A person who, in respect of the offence, has been made the subject of an order under section 210F(1) of the Criminal Procedure (Scotland) Act 1995 (order for lifelong restriction)	An indefinite period beginning with that date
A person who, in respect of the offence or finding, is or has been admitted to a hospital subject to a restriction order	An indefinite period beginning with that date
A person who, in respect of the offence, is or has been sentenced to imprisonment for a term of more than six months but less than 30 months	Ten years beginning with that date
A person who, in respect of the offence, is or has been sentenced to imprisonment for a term of six months or less	Seven years beginning with that date
A person who, in respect of the offence or finding, is or has been admitted to a hospital without being subject to a restriction order	Seven years beginning with that date
A person within section 80(1)(d) (in England and Wales or in Northern Ireland) is cautioned in respect of such an offence	Two years beginning with that date
A person in whose case an order for conditional discharge or, in Scotland, a probation order, is made in respect of the offence	The period of conditional discharge or, in Scotland, the probation period
A person of any other description	Five years beginning with the relevant date

Where a person is under 18 on the relevant date, the period of notification will be one half of the period detailed above. (Crown Copyright)

(In March 2000, a Home Office Circular detailed that 'cautions' no longer exist and are replaced by a 'final warning' and 'reprimand' system. Final warnings and reprimands are equivalent to cautions for the purposes of the Sexual Offences Act 2003.)

A number of aspects exist that may affect the above periods of notification. The Act and all parts pertaining to notification can be obtained from Her Majesty's Stationery Office website: www.legislation.hmso.gov.uk.

The mandatory obligations of a person made subject to notification (Sex Offenders Register)

In brief, a person who has been made subject of a Notification Order will provide the following to the police at a designated police station within three days of the relevant date (conviction or caution or other finding), or release from custody.

Initial notification (registration)

1 The relevant offender's date of birth.
2 His national insurance number.
3 His name on the relevant date and, where he used one or more other names on that date, each of those names.
4 His home address on the relevant date.
5 His name on the date on which notification is given and, where he uses one or more other names on that date, each of those names.
6 His home address on the date on which notification is given.
7 The address of any other premises in the United Kingdom at which, at the time the notification is given, he regularly resides or stays.

Change of personal details

1 A relevant offender must, within the period of three days beginning with:
  a his using a name which has not been notified to the police under section 83(1), this subsection, or section 2 of the Sex Offenders Act 1997 (c. 51)
  b any change of his home address
  c his having resided or stayed, for a qualifying period, at any premises in the United Kingdom the address of which has not been notified to the police under section 83(1), this subsection, or section 2 of the Sex Offenders Act 1997, or
  d his release from custody pursuant to an order of a court or from imprisonment, service detention or detention in a hospital
  notify to the police that name, the new home address, the address of those premises or (as the case may be) the fact that he has been released, and (in addition) the information set out in section 83(5).
2 A notification under subsection (1) may be given before the name is used, the change of home address occurs or the qualifying period ends, but in that case the relevant offender must also specify the date when the event is expected to occur.
3 If a notification is given in accordance with subsection (2) and the event to which it relates occurs more than two days before the date specified, the notification does not affect the duty imposed by subsection (1).
4 If a notification is given in accordance with subsection (2) and the event to which it relates has not occurred by the end of the period of three days beginning with the date specified:
  a the notification does not affect the duty imposed by subsection (1), and
  b the relevant offender must, within the period of six days beginning with the date specified, notify to the police the fact that the event did not occur within the period of three days beginning with the date specified.
5 Section 83(6) applies to the determination of the period of three days mentioned in subsection (1) and the period of six days mentioned in subsection (4)(b), as it applies to the determination of the period mentioned in section 83(1).
6 In this section, 'qualifying period' means:
  a a period of 7 days, or
  b two or more periods, in any period of 12 months, which taken together amount to seven days.

Periodic notification (registration)

1 A relevant offender must, within the period of one year after each event within subsection (2), notify to the police the information set out in section 83(5), unless within that period he has given a notification under section 84(1).

2 The events are:

    a the commencement of this Part (but only in the case of a person who is a relevant offender from that commencement)

    b any notification given by the relevant offender under section 83(1) or 84(1) and

    c any notification given by him under subsection (1).

3 Where the period referred to in subsection (1) would (apart from this subsection) end while subsection (4) applies to the relevant offender, that period is to be treated as continuing until the end of the period of three days beginning when subsection (4) first ceases to apply to him.

4 This subsection applies to the relevant offender if he is:

    a remanded in or committed to custody by an order of a court

    b serving a sentence of imprisonment or a term of service detention

    c detained in a hospital, or

    d outside the United Kingdom.

Foreign travel notification

1 The Secretary of State may by regulations make provision requiring relevant offenders who leave the United Kingdom, or any description of such offenders:

    a to give in accordance with the regulations, before they leave, a notification under subsection (2)

    b if they subsequently return to the United Kingdom, to give in accordance with the regulations a notification under subsection (3).

2 A notification under this subsection must disclose:

    a the date on which the offender will leave the United Kingdom

    b the country (or, if there is more than one, the first country) to which he will travel and his point of arrival (determined in accordance with the regulations) in that country

    c any other information prescribed by the regulations which the offender holds about his departure from or return to the United Kingdom or his movements while outside the United Kingdom.

3 A notification under this subsection must disclose any information prescribed by the regulations about the offender's return to the United Kingdom.

4 Regulations under subsection (1) may make different provision for different categories of person.

Amendments to the Sexual Offences Act or new Acts covering the issue of sexual offences and sexual offenders are accessible via the Home Office website: www.homeoffice.gov.uk.

A brief overview of legislation pertaining to Sexual Offences Prevention Orders (SOPOs) and Risk of Sexual Harm Orders (RSHOs)

(For the purposes of the section, I will refer to the person 'posing risk' as the 'defendant'.)

In addition to Notification Orders, defendants posing risk of significant harm to any other person can be made subject to an order imposed by a court to restrict their activities or behaviour which is deemed to be significantly harmful to another or, by its nature, poses a risk of significant harm to another.

Sexual Offences Prevention Orders (SOPOs)

Criteria for application – upon complaint

The police, Probation Service and the Prison Service are generally the agencies responsible for the management of offenders and persons posing risk to others. Other agencies invariably become involved, such as social services, health department and education welfare, etc. When a defendant is identified, the circumstances are shared between the agencies and decisions are made to implement action which will either reduce or countermand the risk. This process is known as the Multi Agency Public Protection Arrangements (MAPPA). If the participating agencies agree that the service of a SOPO is the most suitable course of action, the police will undertake to consider the application for such an order.

Two specific factors must be in evidence before an application can be considered by a court. They are:

1   that the person is a 'qualifying offender', and
2   that since the 'appropriate date' he has acted in such a way as to give reasonable cause to believe that an order is necessary to protect the public, or any member of the public, from serious sexual harm from him.

Note

A 'qualifying offender' is a person who has been convicted or cautioned for an offence that is listed within Schedule 3 or 5 of the Sexual Offences Act 2003.

An 'appropriate date' relates to the first date on which the defendant was convicted, cautioned or had a finding against him for an offence listed within Schedule 3 or 5 of the Sexual Offences Act 2003. In addition, the most recent concerning act that indicates a posed risk must have occurred within the previous six months to the date upon which the authority (police or other agency) serves a court summons on the person posing the risk.

Applications for SOPOs upon complaint are heard at criminal magistrates courts, although the legislation pertaining to SOPOs is governed in civil law.

Criteria for application – upon conviction

In circumstances where the police are in pursuance of criminal proceedings against a person for committing sexual offences listed in Schedule 3 or 5 of the Sexual Offences Act 2003, consideration should be given to applying to the presiding court for a SOPO. The Crown Prosecution Service, in conjunction with the police, can apply for a SOPO providing that the case and finding are heard at a relevant court and that the defendant receives a relevant custodial sentence.

Note

A 'relevant court', for the purposes of this Act, will be a Crown or a High Court.

A 'relevant custodial sentence' for the purposes of this Act is no less than 12 months.

Applications for SOPOs upon conviction can only be made at Magistrates Court, Crown Court or High Court (depending on criteria) although the legislation pertaining to SOPOs is under civil law.

A SOPO replaces both the Sex Offender Order (Crime and Disorder Act 1998) and the Sex Offender Restraining Order (Criminal Justice and Court Services Act 2000).

A SOPO or Interim SOPO upon service will require the person named thereon to register their personal details with the police as is set out in s83(5) of the Sexual Offences Act 2003 (Notification Requirements).

Restrictions

The whole purpose of Sexual Offences Prevention Orders is to prohibit the defendant from acting in such a way as to allow him to offend or put himself in a position to offend. The restrictions placed upon him must therefore be tailored to suit his offence-threatening activities and provide as great an amount of protection for the public as is possible. However, the restrictions must also be balanced with allowing him to lead as normal a life as is possible and, where achievable, not to negatively impact upon his livelihood.

Only one SOPO can be in force upon a person at any one time and they are imposed for a fixed period of no less than five years from the date of the service of the order, or for an indefinite period.

Risk of Sexual Harm Orders (RSHOs)

Criteria for application

RSHOs were brought into force to deal exclusively with persons posing significant harm to children who had not previously been either convicted or cautioned for any sexual offences or any other offences; and, therefore, will only be applied for 'upon application' and not at the time of any conviction.

With respect to a RSHO, one or more of the acts of significant harm have to fall within the parameters of s.123(3) of the Sexual Offences Act 2003. The acts to which s.123(3) relates are:

1 engaging in sexual activity involving a child or in the presence of a child
2 causing or inciting a child to watch a person engage in sexual activity or to look at a moving or still image that is sexual
3 giving a child anything that relates to a sexual activity or contains reference to such activity
4 communicating with a child, where any part of the communication is sexual.
   It is therefore reasonable to assume that the agencies most likely to identify such persons are the police and social services.

Note

Section 124(5) of the Sexual Offences Act 2003 defines 'sexual activity' as an activity that a reasonable person would, in all the circumstances, but regardless of any person's purpose, consider to be sexual.

Restrictions

As with SOPOs, the whole significance of a RSHO is protection. In the case of RSHOs, the protection is solely concentrated toward children. Restrictions must relate to preventing any acts which would, if not prevented, cause serious physical or psychological harm to a child. The acts concerned must be those detailed in s.123(3) of the Sexual Offences Act 2003 (as outlined above).

Only one RSHO can be in force upon a person at any one time and they are imposed for either a fixed period lasting up to two years, or are indefinite.

Note
1 A Sexual Offences Prevention Order is applicable to persons of any age who pose a risk of significant harm to another of any age.
2 A Risk of Sexual Harm Order is only applicable to persons who have reached 18 years of age and who pose a significant risk of harm to children.

Issues concerning both SOPOs and RSHOs

Interim Orders, variations and renewals

Where a SOPO on application or a RSHO is sought, application can be made to a magistrate's court for an Interim Order to be made. The court can impose an Interim Order if it considers it necessary. There are no guidelines as to the required burden or standard of proof for an Interim Order. The Interim Order will last for a fixed period and will cease to have effect on the date of the finding of an application for a full order.

A variation or renewal of an imposed order can be applied for by the defendant or by the chief constable for the relevant area. Any variation or renewal must contain restrictions that are pertinent to public (children in the case of a RSHO) protection.

Appeals

The defendant may appeal against the making of an order, any variation or renewal. All appeals are made to a Crown Court.

Consequences of breaching a SOPO or an RSHO

If a person who is in receipt of such an order fails to maintain adherence to the restrictions detailed therein, he or she will be considered to have breached the order. If found guilty of such an offence at a criminal court, the defendant concerned may be punishable by way of summary conviction to imprisonment not exceeding six months, a fine or both, but if convicted on indictment, may be sentenced to a term of imprisonment not exceeding five years.

Reference

Office of Public Sector Information: www.opsi.gov.uk

Parents – who to contact

Every teaching establishment has an appointed person or persons responsible for Child Protection – most commonly called an Education Welfare Officer

Every hospital has a Child Protection appointed representative

Your District Council, local police force, GP or school can put you in contact with the people you most need to speak to

Social services departments offer both Child Protection units and counselling

These services are for the victims of abuse and their families

Obvious acts or suspicions of neglect, paedophilia, sexual, emotional, or physical abuse should be reported to

THE POLICE or SOCIAL SERVICES

Useful contact details

Child Protection Organisations

NATIONAL ASSOCIATION FOR THE PREVENTION OF CRUELTY TO CHILDREN (NSPCC)
A telephone helpline for anyone, including children, who has concerns for the welfare of a child or children. This may include persons who are committing child abuse. It is also for persons who are at risk of, or suffering, immediate abuse
Available 24 hours – Tel 0800 800 500

CHILDLINE
Offers telephone counselling and advice to both children and young persons who find themselves in danger or in any kind of trouble
Available 24 hours – Freephone 0800 1111

KIDSCAPE
Provides a free Child Protection leaflet with an SAE and also a telephone helpline for the parents of children suffering bullying
Available 10am–4pm daily – Tel 0207 730 3300

CHILDREN'S LEGAL CENTRE
Advice about the law relating to children in England and Wales
Available 2pm–5pm Mon–Fri – Tel 01206 873820

PARENTLINE PLUS
A telephone helpline for parents who wish to discuss concerns or worries about their child or children
Available 9am–9pm Mon–Fri – Tel 0808 8002222

VICTIM SUPPORT
Offers the victims of crime (abuse either sexual, emotional or neglect) confidential help and advice from highly trained volunteers
Available 24 hours – Tel 0845 30 30 900

SAMARITANS
Offers victims of crime or sufferers of personal tragedy both practical and confidential help and advice from trained and experienced volunteers and staff
Available 24 hours – Tel 0345 909090

CHILD – VICTIMS OF CRIME
Offers children and parents practical help, access to counselling and various other forms of support
www.cvoc.org.uk

INTERNET WATCH FOUNDATION (IWF)
Will investigate any reports of web sites offering or seemingly offering illegal or immoral child abuse material
www.iwf.org.uk

CHILD EXPLOITATION AND ON-LINE PROTECTION (CEOP)
Will investigate any reports of illegal or immoral internet use
www.ceop.gov.uk
General enquiries 0870 000 3344

EVERY CHILD MATTERS (ECM)
Government initiative to increase awareness and support for families and carers with child protection issues, ensuring correct intervention when necessary, and making sure that child protection/care workers are properly trained
www.everychildmatters.gov.uk

The Victoria Climbié Inquiry
Lord Laming's inquiry into the death of Victoria Climbié
www.victoria-climbié-inquiry.org.uk

Glossary

A

Adolescence — The period of life from puberty to maturity terminating legally at the age of sixteen years (UK).

Age of consent — The age at which full civil rights are accorded.

Asexual — An individual lacking sexual attraction and/or romantic feelings towards both sexes.

Assault —
a) A violent physical or verbal attack.
b) A threat or attempt to inflict offensive physical contact or bodily harm on a person that puts the person in immediate danger of or in apprehension of such harm or contact.
c) An assault may be committed without actually touching, or striking, or doing bodily harm, to the person of another.

B

Bisexual — An individual, having both male and female reproductive organs (hermaphroditic), or having a sexual orientation to persons of either sex.

Bondage — Restraining or being restrained in the build-up, during or after the commission of a sexual act.

C

CAI — Child Abuse Images.

Child — Progeny; offspring of parentage. Unborn or recently born human being. In common law one who had not attained the age of 13 years, though the meaning now varies in different statutes; e.g., child labour, support, criminal, and other statutes. Defined within Section 105 of the Children Act 1989, a child is any person under the age of 18 years.

Child (biological) — A child's biological age is not a rate of growth that is actually visible. Biological age is based primarily on "physiological development of the various organs and systems in the body". Examples of organs and systems from which biological age can be determined are bone development, and the efficiency of the heart and lungs to transport oxygen. When biological age is considered with regard to paedophilia, it is with reference to a time preceding puberty.

Child Abuse — Any form of harm or cruelty inflicted on a child that causes a detrimental influence upon its physical, moral, or

	mental well being. This of course includes both contact and non-contact sexual acts.
Child in Need	Where a child whose mental, emotional and physical development may be impaired without the intervention and support of the Local Authority Services, and where no criminal activity is in evidence and no police action taken.
Child Molestation	A common term used to describe a contact sexual act, carried out by an adult upon a child. Child molestation also occurs if the child is forced or coerced into carrying out a contact sexual act upon an adult.
Circumcision	Male circumcision involves the complete or partial removal of the foreskin. Female circumcision involves the removal of the clitoris or its hood and is illegal in most countries.
Cognitive Distortions	MAGNIFICATION OR MINIMISATION: The exaggeration of the importance of things or matters, or to inappropriately understate things or matters until they appear insignificant. To irrationalise the rational or to view a situation or circumstance in such a false way as to see only the positive, the acceptable or the agreeable.
CSA	Child Sexual Abuse.

E

Emergency Protection Order	An Order granted by a magistrate's court to any person applying, with reasonable cause, (usually the Local Authority or DDS), to remove a child from where it is kept if it is likely to suffer significant harm if not removed.
Ephebophile	The term ephebophile refers in principle to an adult who is sexually and emotionally attracted to adolescents (individuals who are younger than eighteen).

F

FII	Fabricated and Induced Illness.
Fixated	To be obsessively interested in, or focused upon a specific.
Forensic Medical	A medical examination where physical and observation evidence is obtained.

G

Gerontophile	A gerontophile is a non-elderly person who possesses a sexual preference or fixation for elderly persons and views them as objects of sexual desire.
Grooming	This word takes on a whole new meaning when used in the context of sexual offender behaviour. 'Grooming' is the process by which an adult with a sexual interest in children will gain control of a child (and where necessary, control of family members) in such a fashion as to be able to sexually abuse a child with little or no concern for the child speaking out and reporting the abuse.

H

Hebephile	An adult who is sexually and emotionally attracted to adolescents (younger than eighteen).
Hermaphrodite	An individual born with both male and female sex organs.
Heterosexism	The belief in an individual's mind, that every person born is heterosexual by default; and that heterosexuality is the superior, or only true sexual orientation.
Heterosexual	An individual who is sexually orientated to persons of the opposite sex (gender).
Homophobia	An extreme aversion to homosexuality and homosexual people.
Homosexual	An individual who is sexually orientated to persons of the same sex (gender).

I

IIG	Internet Initiated Grooming.
Intrafamilial	A word meaning 'within the family'.

J

Juvenile	A young person (a period of one's life when one is young; in particular: the period between childhood and maturity).

K

Korophilia	A descriptive word for those who possess the love of, or are attracted to young men or boys.

L

Lesbian	A woman whose sexual orientation is to women.

M

Masturbation	The self stimulation of one's sexual organs.
Maternal	Motherly; relating to or characteristic features of motherhood.
Minor	A person who has not attained the age of consent.

N

Necrophilia	Used to describe an erotic fascination or obsession with the dead. For some, sexual arousal can be generated by the sight or odour of a corpse. The word also describes an act whereby an individual copulates with a corpse.
Nepiophilia	Also called infantophilia. This term describes adults who are sexually attracted to 'babies' or 'infants'.

O

Orgasm	The peak of sexual excitement, characterised by strong feelings of pleasure and by a series of involuntary contractions of the muscles of the genitals, usually accompanied by the ejaculation of sperm by the male. Also called *climax*.

P

Paederasty	A word describing sexual activity involving a man and a boy.
Paediatrician	A medical reference to one who is a specialist in the care of babies and young children.
Paedophile	One affected by paedophilia.
Paedophilia	A sexual orientation of an adult (male or female) who is emotionally and/or sexually attracted to pre-pubescent children.
Pansexual	An individual who possesses all sexual orientations.
Paraphilia	A term often used to describe one of a number of sexual preferences in which an adult's sexual arousal or sexual fantasy consists of sexual activity involving either non-human objects, children or adolescents, other non-consenting individuals, or the infliction of pain upon another.
Parental-Responsibility	Legal stance – Children ACT 1989 A responsibility held by either the natural mother, the natural father if the child's parents were married at the of the child's birth, the natural father if a parental responsibility agreement has been drawn up in the form prescribed by the Lord Chancellor, or any person having parental responsibility by virtue of some form of court order (Sections 2 and 4 of the Children Act 1989).
Partner	A socially and politically correct term to describe one's heterosexual or homosexual lover, significant other, boyfriend or girlfriend on a public level.
Paternal	Fatherly; relating to or characteristic features of fatherhood.
Police Protection	A lawful Power under Section 46 of the Children Act 1989, allowing a constable who has reasonable cause to believe that a child would otherwise be likely to suffer significant harm to: • remove a child to suitable accommodation and keep her or him there • take such steps as are reasonable to ensure that the child's removal from any hospital, or other place in which she or he is then being accommodated, is prevented.
POLIT	Police On-Line Investigation Team.
Puberty	Is the period in a human's life in which physical growth and sexual maturation occurs.

R

Rape	Unlawful sexual intercourse with a male or female (sexual intercourse without consent).
Referral	A documented record of information supplied to either the Social Services Department or Police, outlining the welfare or concerns regarding one or more children.

Regression	The action or an act of falling back, to retire, relapse or degenerate; or regressing to an earlier stage of life or a supposed previous life.

S

Sadism-Masochism (S&M)	Sadism: Inflicting pain on others for sexual gratification. Masochism: Receiving pain and/or humiliation for sexual gratification.
Scatophilia	The obtaining of sexual pleasure by way of making obscene telephone calls or other communicating.
Scoptophilia	The obtaining of sexual pleasure by covertly watching another person undress or have sex – often referred to as 'voyeurism'.
Sex Offender	An individual who has been convicted of any offence pertaining to sexual matters. These include contact and non-contact sexual offences.
Sex Offender Registration	The recording of the personal details by the police, of individuals who have been convicted of one or more specific sexual offences.
Sexual Orientation	Sexual orientation is psychological. It is one's mental view of the 'sexual ideal'. In short: 'the gender, age range and physical appearance of another, to which one is emotionally and sexually attracted and aroused'.
Significant Harm	A situation which is life threatening or traumatic and from which recovery, whether physical or psychological, can be expected to be difficult or impossible.
Sodomy	Anal penetrative sexual intercourse committed by a man with a man or woman.
STD	Sexually Transmitted Disease.

T

Transgendered/ Transsexual	Individuals, either heterosexual or homosexual, who are more comfortable portraying a member of the opposite sex; or who complete a sex (gender) change.
Transvestite	A man, either heterosexual or homosexual, who derives pleasure from dressing as a woman.

U

USI	Unlawful Sexual Intercourse: this occurs when and adult has sexual intercourse with a minor who is a willing participant, but legally, cannot give consent. Now detailed in law as Indecent Sexual Assault by Penetration.
UTI	Urinary Tract Infection.

X

Xenophobic	A descriptive word for a person who is unduly fearful or has a hatred for that which is foreign, especially of strangers or foreign peoples.

Z

Zoophilia	A love of non-human animals.

Index